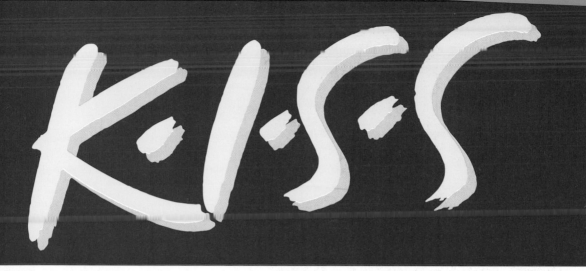

K·I·S·S

GUIDE TO

Weight Loss

BARBARA RAVAGE

Foreword by **Kathy Smith**
America's leading fitness expert

A Dorling Kindersley Book

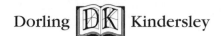
Dorling **DK** Kindersley

LONDON, NEW YORK, SYDNEY, DELHI, PARIS,
MUNICH, AND JOHANNESBURG

Dorling Kindersley Publishing, Inc.

Editorial Director: LaVonne Carlson
Series Editor: Jennifer Williams
Senior Editor: Jill Hamilton
Editor: Joseph Gonzales
Copyeditors: Jim Lubin, Matthew Kiernan

Dorling Kindersley Limited

Category Publisher: Mary Thompson
Managing Editor: Maxine Lewis
Managing Art Editor: Heather McCarry
Project Editor: David Tombesi-Walton
Project Art Editors: Justin Clow, Simon Murrell
Jacket Designer: Neal Cobourne
Picture Researchers: Melanie Simmonds, Marcus Scott
Production: Heather Hughes

Produced for Dorling Kindersley by **Cooling Brown**
9–11 High Street, Hampton, Middlesex TW12 2SA

Creative Director: Arthur Brown
Art Editor: Hilary Krag
Senior Editor: Amanda Lebentz
Editors: Mary Lambert, Alison Bolus

Library of Congress Cataloging-in-Publication Data

Ravage, Barbara.
   KISS guide to weight loss / Barbara Ravage.-- 1st American ed.
      p. cm. -- (Keep it simple series)
   Includes index.
     ISBN 0-7894-6139-0 (alk. paper)
     1. Weight loss. I. Title. II. Series.
RM222.2 . R375 2000
613.7--dc21

00-010801

Dorling Kindersley Publishing, Inc. offers special discounts for bulk purchases for sales promotions or premiums.
Specific, large-quantity needs can be met with special editions, including personalized covers,
excerpts of existing guides, and corporate imprints. For more information, contact Special Markets Department,
Dorling Kindersley Publishing, Inc., 95 Madison Avenue, New York, NY 10016 Fax: 800-600-9098.

Color reproduction by ColourScan, Singapore
Printed and bound by Printer Industria Grafica, S.A., Barcelona, Spain

For our complete catalog visit

www.dk.com

Contents at a Glance

CONTENTS

PART ONE *Thinking About It*

CHAPTER 1 Are You Overweight?   22

CHAPTER 2 Why Lose Weight?   38

PART THREE Looking At Yourself

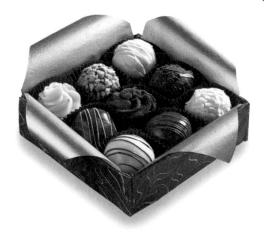

PART FIVE Doing It

PART SIX Keeping It Up

APPENDICES

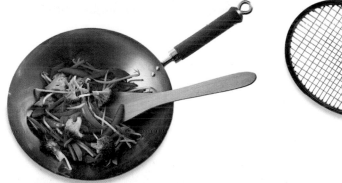
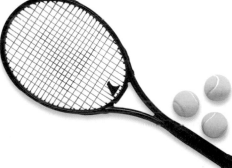

Foreword

5/5/03

WE ALL WANT TO BE BEAUTIFUL. *It's human nature to admire what's beautiful and aspire to it. And our drive to seek beauty is a good one: It can motivate us to take care of ourselves, pursue better health, and create more harmony in our surroundings. But when the drive for glamour is taken to the extreme, we can lose sight of what is truly beautiful. We are constantly barraged by images of people with perfect skin, slim figures, and youthful glows. While these people look lovely, we must keep reminding ourselves not to compare ourselves to them (or anyone else for that matter). Each of us, as individuals, must strive to find our own personal definition of beauty.*

True beauty, I believe, begins with our feelings about ourselves – inside and out. Finding the right balance of good food, enjoyable exercise, and a healthy dose of self-confidence will contribute to a feeling of well-being. If you are already including these good habits in your life, congratulations! But if you don't like what you see when you look around, then it's time for a change.

Weight loss can be an important part of getting to that point where you feel good about who you are. Carrying less weight may help you move more gracefully, feel healthier, and release some of that society-induced guilt about "being overweight." But what's really important is the realization that weight loss is not your ultimate goal – it's a step toward getting where you want to be.

Building a strong foundation on the physical side can go a long way toward helping you feel good. Eating well, exercising regularly, and establishing healthy habits can do a lot to keep you feeling great. _As you continue to develop better habits, you gain the confidence you need to keep yourself going, even when temptation – or just plain tiredness – may strike._

As good as you may feel about watching your weight and staying fit, you're likely to need an occasional guide. That guide can come in many forms: a close friend who acts as a personal cheerleader; an upbeat video that helps you over that low-energy hump; and an accessible book that gives you practical information to keep you on the right track. This K.I.S.S. Guide to Weight Loss can do just that, so you'll be less tempted to follow the newest – but not necessarily the safest – food fads. This guide can help you assess where you're at, what you can reasonably expect to achieve, and how to get there safe and sound.

After all, true fitness – like true beauty – comes from within. Finding that inner beauty begins with your awareness of the close connection between being healthy and feeling good. Sharing that beauty comes when you put that awareness into practice and become the person you've always aspired to be. I wish you all the best on your journey toward true, inner fitness.

Kathy Smith

KATHY SMITH
AMERICA'S LEADING FITNESS EXPERT

Introduction

WEIGHT LOSS IS A $33 BILLION INDUSTRY. *There are literally thousands of books and videos on diet and exercise. On every newsstand, you can find magazines by the dozens featuring weight-loss stories on their covers. The World Wide Web is bloated with information on the subject. Mail order catalogues are fat with supplements, potions, preparations, and devices that "guarantee" a trimmer, firmer you.*

The shelves of your corner drugstore and health food emporium are groaning with similar products. There are diet plan purveyors and exercise gurus who want you to trade pounds for dollars. The medical profession has weighed in with prescription drugs, medically supervised diets, and surgery ranging from liposuction to stomach staples. Hypnotism, acupuncture, magnets, and herbs are touted as new ways to fight the urge to overeat. Support groups offer support, gyms and recreational centers are equipped with weight machines and exercise classes. If there's a penny to be made on the American obsession with weight, someone will surely find it. Many already have.

One way to look at this glut of information and products is that it fills a need: Americans in general are overweight and most of us want to do something about it. Another way to see it is that if there were any single answer to this weighty issue, all we'd need is a single, one-diet-fits-all approach.

But what is a person to do? How can you figure out whether you need to lose weight, and if so, how much? And most important of all, how can you figure out the most effective way to do it?

That's where the K.I.S.S. Guide to Weight Loss comes in. The book you hold in your hand will provide you with a simple map for navigating the murky waters of weight loss. But be warned: If you're looking for a quick fix, a magic bullet, an easy way, you've picked up the wrong book. Because the simple truth is there is no easy way.

Let this be your motto: "If it's fast, it won't last."

I'm interested in what will last, and if you are too, we'll get along fine. Step by step, we'll take a look at how far your real body is from your ideal, and figure out how to get you as close to that ideal as is possible. More important, we'll figure out how to keep you there once you've arrived.

I'll begin by showing you a simple way to determine whether you are overweight or have other problems with food that are interfering with your health. Next you'll learn a bit about why weighing too much is not healthy. I'll debunk some popular myths about eating and weight loss, and give you the solid facts. And finally, we'll look at the real way to lose weight:

- *Reduce your calorie intake by eating sensibly;*
- *Increase your calorie output with regular exercise;*
- *Modify your behavior to develop lifelong healthy eating and exercise habits.*

Along the way, I'll help you identify and understand your problem behaviors related to eating and exercise. Together we'll work out a simple plan that suits you – not your neighbor who lost 30 pounds in one month (and has probably gained it all back by now); not the movie star who had her fat surgically redistributed; and not the supermodel who subsists on wheat grass and diet soda. But you, the flesh-and-blood person who simply wants to be as healthy as possible to get the fullest enjoyment out of life!

BARBARA RAVAGE

What's Inside?

THE INFORMATION in the K.I.S.S. Guide to Weight Loss *is arranged so that you can think and learn about weight issues, plan a weight-loss program to suit you, lose the pounds you want to, and keep them off – for good.*

PART ONE

In Part One I'll help you to assess whether or not you are overweight, look at the effects of being overweight, and investigate how fitness (or lack of it) affects the body.

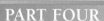

PART TWO

In Part Two I'll take you through the basics of nutrition, explain why calories are so important and give you straight answers to some frequently asked weight-loss questions.

PART THREE

In Part Three I'll be asking *you* to question your attitudes about food and to review your own fitness. Then we'll start thinking about what you want to achieve in the future.

PART FOUR

In Part Four I'll show you how to plan for success: how to avoid pitfalls, adopt diet-smart strategies, start an exercise program, and plan your daily calorie intake.

PART FIVE

In Part Five I'll talk tactics: how to stay motivated on your weight-loss program, live happily with your diet, and get the most from your exercise routine.

PART SIX

In Part Six I'll focus on how keep up your plan and integrate it into your daily life. I'll also show you ways to overcome common obstacles, so whether you're dreading eating out, you've lapsed, or you're bored, you'll find troubleshooting tips here.

The Extras

THROUGHOUT THE BOOK, *you'll find four different types of icons scattered throughout the text. They're meant to make life simpler for the browser by acting as road signs, drawing your attention to specific types of information. Here are the icons and what they mean:*

Very Important Point

Don't eat . . . I mean, read another word until you've digested these items.

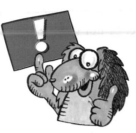

✓

Complete No-No

These are warnings about things that may be dangerous or unhealthy or may just doom your efforts to failure.

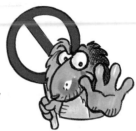

✓

Getting Technical

If the experts know it, why shouldn't you? If you like knowing how things work and why, pay attention. If you're not interested, just move on.

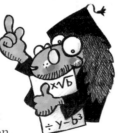

✓

Inside Scoop

Inside information and tips from the pros that will help you reach your goal.

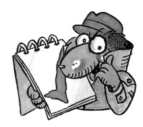

✓

Throughout the text, you'll also find three different types of boxes containing helpful tips and extra information to smooth your path to weight loss.

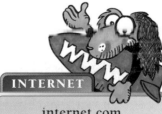

Trivia...
If you like odd little facts, these tidbits may lighten the burden of losing weight.

✓

DEFINITION
*I'll try not to use confusing or unfamiliar terms, but if you run across one in the text, you'll find the term **explained** in a box right on the same page.*

✓

INTERNET
internet.com
If your favorite exercise is surfing the Internet, you'll find more information on the topics we've discussed at the Web addresses listed in these boxes.

✓

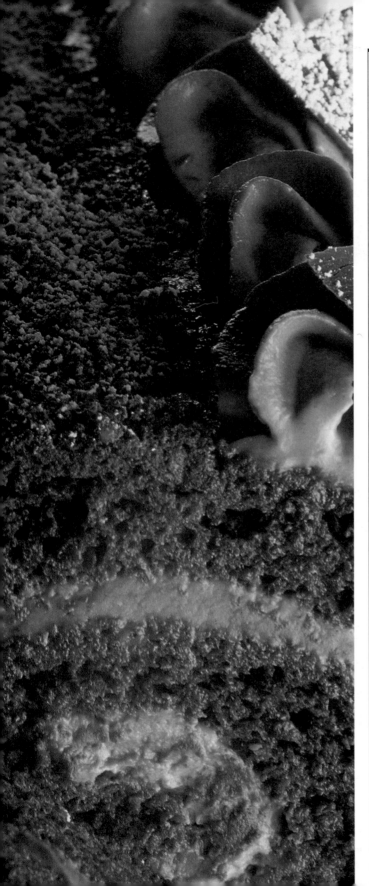

PART ONE

CHOCOLATE CAKE: TEMPTING BUT CALORIE-LADEN

THINKING ABOUT IT

YOU'VE PROBABLY BEEN THINKING about losing weight for a while, maybe because you know you're *overweight* 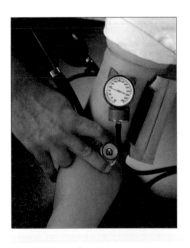 or only because you think you are. Most likely, you've been down this road before. You may have succeeded in losing some or all of the weight you wanted to shed, but not in keeping it off. Or maybe you have tried and failed to lose more than a few pounds.

Whatever your situation, we are all in the same boat. Gaining weight is easy: All you have to do is eat. Losing weight is hard. And keeping it off is even harder. Some experts say it is as hard as kicking drug addiction or quitting smoking. And like these two efforts, losing excess weight is critical to your *health* and *well-being*. At the end of Part One, I hope you will be thinking about weight loss in a new way, in a way that works for you.

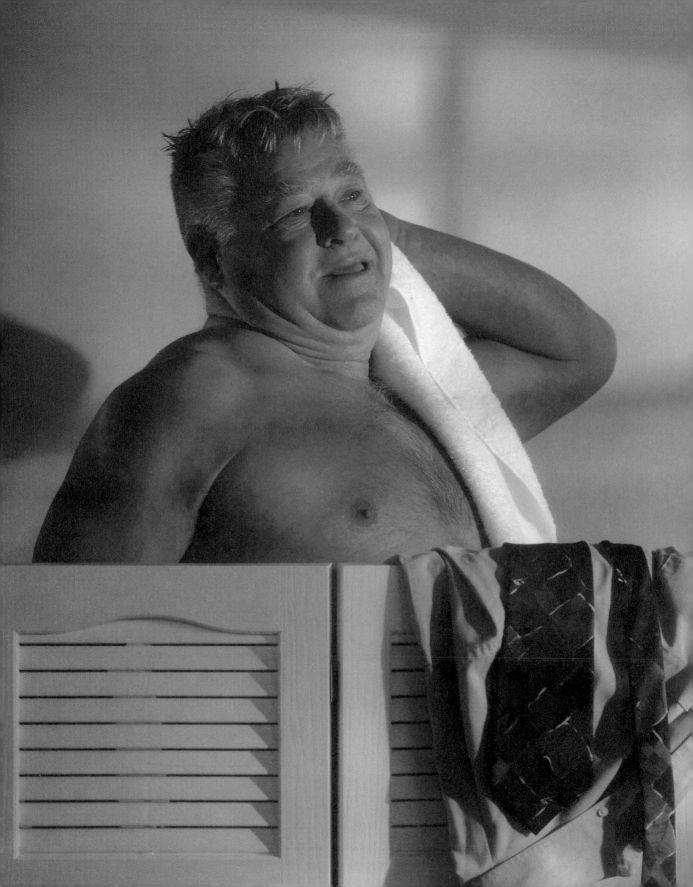

Chapter 1

Are You Overweight?

Y OU THINK YOU NEED to lose some weight, otherwise you wouldn't be reading this book. But do you really need to slim down? Before embarking on a weight-loss effort, it's a good idea to focus on what your personal challenge will be. This chapter will give you the tools to collect the data you need and to design a weight-loss program that will work for you.

In this chapter...

✓ Before you begin

✓ What is overweight?

✓ More body fat measures

✓ Working it all out

✓ Talk to your doctor

✓ Look in the mirror

✓ Ask your family and friends

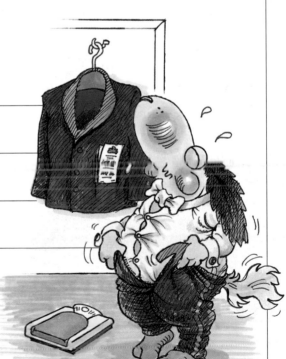

Before you begin

THIS BOOK WILL FOCUS on you. Not on a weight-loss fantasy and not on what might work for your next-door neighbor. That means I'll be asking you some very personal questions and expecting you to write down the answers. So the first step is to get a notebook.

Buy a notebook that will inspire you. ✓ ~~Notebook~~

Your notebook might simply be a loose-leaf binder to which you can add pages photocopied from this book or material printed out from the many Internet resources I'll be telling you about. You might prefer something small enough to slip into your purse or gym bag. The pages of your notebook can be lined, blank, or ruled like graph paper. It could have a pretty cover or a blank one on which you can tape pictures that will motivate you. The important thing is that the notebook should be devoted exclusively to your weight-loss project. Do not use it for any other purpose.

Your personal database

Begin at the beginning, with page one of your personal database. This will show you where you were on the first day of the rest of your life. Don't write anything down yet. First you need to understand the territory we'll be exploring together. After that, we'll turn the spotlight on you and do the math together.

What is overweight?

In 1998, the National Institutes of Health released new guidelines for what is considered normal weight, overweight, and obesity. The guidelines are based on body mass index (BMI), which is a ratio between height and weight that fairly accurately reflects the proportion of fat to muscle and other tissues in the body.

According to the guidelines, a BMI between 20 and 24.9 is normal. BMIs between 25 and 29.9 are defined as overweight. And 30 or over is considered obese.

DEFINITION

Body mass index (BMI) is a formula used to estimate the proportion of your body that consists of fat. The formula is weight (kg) ÷ height² (m).

BODY MASS INDEX

Find your BMI on this chart by looking for your height and weight and locating the box where the two columns meet. Or you can calculate your BMI manually by multiplying your weight in pounds by 704, then dividing by the square of your height in inches. For example, if you weigh 162 pounds and are 69 inches (5 ft 9 ins) tall, your BMI is (162 x 704) ÷ (69 x 69) = 23.9. If you use the metric system, divide your weight in kilograms by the square of your height in meters. Refer to the key below to see how you shape up.

Height (in)

Weight (lb)	58	60	62	64	66	68	70	72	74	76	78	Weight (kg)
340	71	66	62	58	55	52	49	46	44	41	39	154
320	67	62	59	55	52	49	46	43	41	39	37	145
300	63	59	55	51	48	46	43	41	39	37	35	136
280	59	55	51	48	45	43	40	38	36	34	32	127
260	54	51	48	45	42	40	37	35	33	32	30	118
240	50	47	44	41	39	36	34	33	31	29	28	109
220	46	43	40	38	36	33	32	30	28	27	25	100
200	42	39	37	34	32	30	29	27	26	24	23	90
180	38	35	33	31	29	27	26	24	23	22	21	82
160	33	31	29	27	26	24	23	22	21	19	18	73
140	29	27	26	24	23	21	20	19	18	17	16	63
120	25	23	22	21	19	18	17	16	15	15	14	54
100	21	20	18	17	16	15	14	14	13	12	12	45
80	17	16	15	14	13	12	11	11	10	10	9	36

| | 147 | 152 | 157 | 163 | 168 | 173 | 178 | 183 | 188 | 193 | 198 | |

Height (cm)

(Handwritten notes in margin: 12/16/02, 5/20/03, GOAL)

KEY

COLOR	BMI	
	Less than 18	Underweight
	18 – 24	Desirable weight
	25 – 29	Overweight
	30 – 40	Obese
	More than 40	Severely obese

Are we getting fatter or have the rules changed?

The answer to both questions is yes. The federal Centers for Disease Control, the U.S. Surgeon General, and numerous public health and research centers have been screaming loudly that we, as a nation, are way too fat. Over the past 20 years, the number of children and adults who are overweight has ballooned. Given the many health problems associated with overweight, this is a major health crisis.

At the same time, the standard for normal weight has been revised downward. Previously, BMIs of 25 and 26 were considered normal, with 27 being the cutoff point. Now the cutoff is 25. This might seem unfair, but it is based on sound medical evidence.

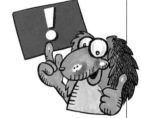

Fair or not, according to the newest guidelines, 55 percent of all Americans are overweight or obese. No doubt about it, weight problems are epidemic in this country!

More body fat measures

BMI IS A PRETTY GOOD WAY to tell whether a person is overweight, but it's an approximate measure that doesn't take into account how muscular you are. Because muscle tissue weighs more than fat, trim and muscular people might weigh enough to put them into the overweight or even obese category. If you are reading this book, we probably aren't talking about you, but I just thought I'd mention it. Conversely, people with very small frames and light bones might fall into the normal range even if they have too much stored fat around the waist and hips.

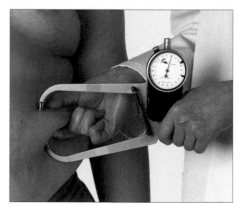

■ **One way of** *telling how much body fat you are carrying is to go for a skinfold test, where calipers are used to measure the thickness of the fat layer under the skin.*

There are some fairly high-tech and expensive ways to measure the proportion of fat in a person's body.

One technique that theoretically can make a distinction between muscle and fat involves being weighed underwater. In another method that "knows" the difference between fat and lean, a harmless electric current is passed through the body. Finally, the skinfold test uses calipers to measure how much fat there is under the skin. It's really just a more professional version of the old "can you pinch an inch?" test.

Height-weight table

Before BMI, people gauged their weight according to a height-weight table that was put out by the Metropolitan Life Insurance Company. The table gave a normal weight range for different heights and frame sizes. There were a number of problems with the table, the biggest being that it was based on insurance company statistics about average weight, rather than on medical evidence about what is healthy and what is not. This measure of normal weight is no longer considered reliable, but it may be useful as a supplement to BMI, as we shall see.

Body type

ACTION

When it comes to health, it turns out that where you carry extra weight matters almost as much as how much you are carrying. This is where the waist-to-hip ratio (WHR = waist÷hip measurement) comes in. A simple way of looking at WHR is to think of body types as apples or pears. Apple types are wide around the waist and abdomen; pears are heavy in the hips, thighs, and buttocks. There's good news and bad news about each type.

For apples, the good news is that they tend to have an easier time losing their "spare tire" once they begin eating sensibly and exercising regularly. The bad news is that they are at greater risk for cardiovascular disease, high blood pressure, diabetes, and some cancers.

> *Trivia...*
> *Who are fatter, women or men? According to the latest National Health and Nutrition Examination Survey, approximately 63 percent of men and 55 percent of women over 25 years of age in the United States. are overweight. When it comes to obesity, though, women are the leaders, with 21 percent of men and 27 percent of women falling into this category. Obviously, there are no winners in the battle of the bulge.*

For pears, the good news is that they are less likely to suffer from heart problems. The bad news is that they are less successful shedding their extra padding.

> *Ideally, women should have a waist-to-hip ratio of 0.8 or less, and men should aim for 0.95 or less.*

In the next section, you'll learn how to figure out your WHR and find out if you're an apple or a pear.

Working it all out

ENOUGH THEORY. Let's get down to brass tacks. It's time to take out your notebook and take off your clothes.

Now you can actually take out that notebook, binder, or folder you bought. Open your book and let's get started with compiling your own personal database. Opposite is an example of how it might look, but you can modify it to suit your taste. You may not be familiar with all the terms in the chart just yet, but you will be by the end of the chapter. Throughout this chapter and those to come, you'll be filling in the blanks.

How much do you weigh?

First step: Get on the scale. I hope you have one.

It's important to have a <u>reliable scale</u>, but that doesn't mean you have to spend a lot of money to buy one or put off thinking about losing weight because you don't have one.

■ **Buy a reliable scale** *if you don't already have one. Weigh yourself (naked) at the same time of day, ideally just once a week, for an accurate record of the pounds you are losing.*

If you have a doctor's balance scale, great. That's the most accurate type. If you have a regular home scale that's fairly new, chances are it is accurate. If you don't have a scale, or one you trust, buy the best you can afford.

The main thing is to always weigh yourself on the same scale and at the <u>same time</u> of day.

That way, even if the weight you get isn't the same as at your doctor's office or gym, it will reflect in relative terms where you began and the distance, pounds-wise, you've traveled.

Take a look at the numbers. Wiggle around a bit if you think it will help, but as soon as the pointer stops moving, write the figure in your personal database.

ACTION

My personal database

Date	✓	10/1			
My weight	✓	200 lbs			
My height	✓	5 ft 4in	➝		
My BMI (body mass index)	✓	34.3			
My ideal weight range	✓	107–147	➝		
Number of pounds more than ideal weight	✓	53 lbs			

MY BODY TYPE

Waist size	✓	40 in			
Hips size	✓	46 in			
My waist-to-hip ratio (WHR)	✓	0.86			

I am an apple or (pear) (circle one) ✓

My main body type problem is: (circle one)

I am at higher risk for diabetes, high blood pressure, heart disease

(Losing weight and keeping it off may be harder for me)

MY MEASUREMENTS

Chest/bust	✓	38 in			
Upper thigh	✓	21 in			
Calf	✓	14 in			
Upper arm	✓	14 in			
Lower arm	✓	10 in			

■ **Use the first page** of your personal database to record all your current measurements. Throughout this chapter, you'll be learning how to do this so that you can plot your way to weight-loss success — and keep track of just how much you've achieved.

How tall are you?

No, there's no way this book can make you taller, but since you will need to know your height to figure out your BMI and find yourself on the height-weight table, you may as well measure yourself. Don't rely on what you think your height has always been. I have spent the better part of my adult life thinking I was 5-foot-nothing, but a few years ago I went to a new doctor, who measured me and informed me that I am 5ft 1in. Maybe I grew in my 40s, who knows? But it did mean I could get away with weighing a bit more before I had to call myself overweight.

The best way to measure your height at home is to stand against a wall in bare feet, with your shoulders back and head straight. Have someone slide a pencil across your scalp and make a mark on the wall. If you're on your own, make a mark yourself, being careful not to hunch your shoulders or move your head. Measure from the floor to the mark on the wall with a tape measure, then add the answer to your personal database.

INTERNET

www.thriveonline.com
/weight/tools/bmi.html

The Internet is full of interactive BMI calculators. This one will not only figure out your BMI for you, but will also give you recommendations on what to do about the result.

What's your BMI?

Take a look at the BMI chart on page 25. Find your height and weight, and locate the number where the two come together. Write your BMI in your personal database.

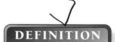

DEFINITION

Body dysphoria *is a psychological condition in which a person has a false sense of his or her own body, often feeling fat when the opposite is true. Many people suffering from anorexia have this false sense of what they look like.*

- Is it under 20? You may be underweight.

If your BMI is under 20 and you think you're fat, do not embark on a weight-loss program without talking with your doctor. There's a strong possibility that you suffer from body dysphoria rather than being overweight

- Is it under 25? That means your weight is normal.

- Is it close to 25? You are right on the border between normal weight and overweight. In your case, regular exercise and sensible eating can help you lose some pounds, get fit, and keep you on the safe side of the BMI table.

- Is it 25 or over? If so, you are overweight and need to do something about it.

- Is it over 30? If so, you are obese.

If your BMI is over 30, you are a higher risk for many health problems, as you will learn in Chapter 2. You may already have one or more disorders or conditions that not only threaten your health, but may require special strategies for diet and exercise. I want you to succeed. I do not want you to further harm your health by following a dangerous diet.

What's your body type?

Are you an apple or a pear? Take off your clothes (unless you didn't get dressed again after weighing yourself) and take out your tape measure. (A cloth or Mylar tape works best when measuring curves.) Measure your waist and write down the measurement in your notebook. Can't find your waist? If you're a serious apple, you may not be familiar with the location of your waist. No, it's not where your pants ride or where you buckle your belt. It's right above your navel and below your ribcage.

If you can, have someone help you measure your height

Measure the waist between ribcage and navel

Here's how to locate your waist: Bend forward or to the side. The place that creases is where your natural waist is

Now measure your hips. Be sure to pass the tape around the widest part of your buttocks. Write down the measurement in your notebook.

Now divide your waist measurement by your hip measurement. That's right, you may be dividing a smaller number by a larger number. Write the answer you get in the space provided in your personal database.

The widest part of the buttocks marks the hips

Is your WHR less than 1? If so, you are a pear. If your WHR is 1 or more, you are an apple. Circle your fruit. Check your personal database for the special problems associated with your body type and circle the one that applies to you.

■ **To find out** *your waist-to-hip ratio and determine whether you are an apple or pear shape, first measure your height. Then divide your waist measurement by your hip measurement.*

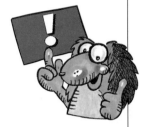

Knowing whether you are an apple or a pear is valuable information, but it doesn't tell you whether you are overweight or not. You may be a small apple, or a very large pear!

Where are you on the height-weight table?

Even though the height-weight table is a less accurate measure of normal and overweight, some people prefer to use it. For one thing, it gives a range of normal weight, and some people like that wiggle room. Instead of using the life insurance company table, which requires you to know your frame size, we'll use a much simpler one that comes from the U.S. Department of Agriculture. Find your height and look at the column for your age range in the table below. You'll see a range of 20 or so pounds for "healthy weight." Women should be on the lighter side, men on the heavier. Write this range in your personal database in the space for "My ideal weight range."

HEIGHT-WEIGHT TABLE

Height	Weight in pounds	
	19 to 34 years	**35 years and over**
5 ft 0 in	97–128	108–138
5 ft 1 in	101–132	111–143
5 ft 2 in	104–137	115–148
5 ft 3 in	107–141	119–152
5 ft 4 in	111–146	122–157
5 ft 5 in	114–150	126–162
5ft 6 in	118–155	130–167
5 ft 7 in	121–160	134–172
5 ft 8 in	125–164	138–178
5 ft 9 in	129–169	142–183
5 ft 10 in	132–174	146–188
5 ft 11 in	136–179	151–194
6 ft 0 in	140–184	155–199
6 ft 1 in	144–189	159–205
6 ft 2 in	148–195	164–210
6 ft 3 in	152–200	168–216
6 ft 4 in	156–205	173–222
6 ft 5 in	160–211	177–228
6 ft 6 in	164–216	182–234

INTERNET

www.iVillage.com/diet/tools/healthcalc/

Another simple way to find out if you are within the normal range for your height, gender, and frame size can be found on this site.

Talk to your doctor

HAS A DOCTOR *ever advised you to lose weight? Has a doctor ever advised you to exercise more? Have you ever been given specific advice or counseling on how to do this?*

Chances are, even if the answer to the first two questions is yes, the answer to the third is no. No less an august publication than the *Journal of the American Medical Association* says that doctors are doing a lousy job of counseling their patients about weight loss and exercise. Even though the National Institutes of Health urged health care professionals to advise their obese patients to lose weight, fewer than half of obese adults report hearing that advice from their doctors. And that's only obese patients. How many people who are merely overweight receive counseling and advice during a doctor visit?

The fact is, you may know more than your doctor about food and fitness. A course in nutrition is required in fewer than 23 percent of medical and dental schools in the United States.

Find a doctor who will help

Some years ago, during my annual physical, I told my doctor I wanted to lose some weight. He reached into his desk drawer, pulled out a single sheet of paper, and slid it across the desk, saying "You look fine to me, but you can try this if you want." The sheet had a week's

■ **Speak frankly** *to your doctor about your weight worries – it's important that you get full support during any weight-loss campaign. If you don't feel that you are being taken seriously, consider changing doctors.*

worth of menus for what I assume was a reduced-calorie diet. Needless to say, that didn't exactly motivate me to lose weight, and I did not.

Three years ago, I switched doctors. (The "weight-loss counseling" I had received was only part of the reason.) My new doctor asked if there were any specific issues I wanted to discuss, and I said I felt fat and depressed. He stopped, paid attention, and asked me if I thought the two were separate issues or part of the same thing. I said I thought maybe a little of both.

He asked me about my exercise habits, which at the time were pretty pathetic. "I walk a lot," I volunteered hopefully. Then he gave me some very specific advice and said he thought it would help lift both burdens. It worked! Not only did I lose 16 pounds over the course of 6 months, but I have kept the weight off for 3 whole years. And although I am sometimes sad, I have not felt really depressed in a very long time.

The reason I tell this story is to show the range of experiences we may have when we talk to our doctors about weight. I was lucky the second time, but I fear my first experience was more typical.

It's important to enlist your doctor in your weight-loss campaign.

Talking to your doctor is especially important if you are very overweight or have weight-related and other health problems, and certainly if you are pregnant. Talk to your doctor before starting on any diet to be sure there is no risk of malnutrition, vitamin deficiency, alterations in your body chemistry, or dangerously rapid weight loss.

Your doctor can be one of your most effective boosters as you work to become healthier. If he or she is not, speak up frankly. Tell your doctor that this is very important to you and that you really need help and concrete advice. If necessary, schedule a separate appointment to discuss your weight and what to do about it. Let your doctor know, in advance, that's the reason you are coming in. And if you still don't get the support and solid information you need, consider changing doctors.

Look in the mirror

YOU PROBABLY DO THIS A LOT ALREADY, *and probably with a certain amount of disgust. This time, think of it as a way to take a good hard look at the problem and analyze it with a view toward the solution. Give yourself some time and privacy in front of a full-length mirror. Look at yourself both dressed and undressed, and from all angles.*

Start a new page in your notebook. Call it "My Body" or "Mirror, Mirror" or whatever works for you. Write down what you see.

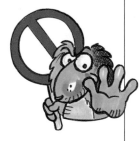

Do not write a totally negative list of everything you hate about your body. Put down some good points as well.

Write down what you like about your body as well as what you don't like, otherwise the list will be too negative and will discourage rather than motivate you. What parts of your body are okay, or nearly okay? Work out where the problem spots are. Does your look change when you change your posture?

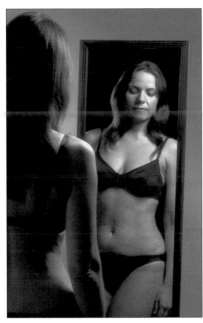

Next write down what you'd like to see. Are you slender in your lower arms, but chunky above the elbows? Are your ankles nice and slim but your thighs puckery? Do you like your cheekbones but wish you had just one chin rather than two? Are your biceps your strong point, but your beer belly an embarrassment?

Change of clothes

Next, put on some clothes that you think work for you. If front-pleated slacks make you look like Bozo the Clown, try on some with a flat front. If you can't button that blazer, maybe a jacket with a boxier cut is more flattering. Was it hard to find something that really fits?

■ **When you look at yourself** in the mirror, study the different parts of your body and note down the good points that you see, as well as the bad.

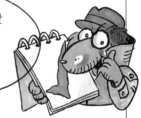

Are there clothes hanging in your closet that you really love but haven't been able to wear? Hang those outfits front and center to remind you what you're aiming toward.

What about the kinds of clothes you love the look of but wouldn't even consider buying? Personally, I have always longed to wear one of those classic sweater dresses, a clingy bit of cashmere or lamb's wool that says "sleek and chic" to me. I admire women who can wear these things and occasionally I'll try one on, telling myself that I'll buy the first one that looks good on me, no matter what the price. Alas, I've never found that perfect dress, and maybe I never will. Still, it's a sort of weight-loss Holy Grail for me, and dreaming about it helps to keep me on track.

Motivation is equal parts dream and reality. Looking in the mirror is your reality check, but it can also help you dream.

Ask your family and friends

TALKING TO PEOPLE *who love you and whom you trust is another way to do a reality check. Ask them whether they think you look too heavy. And then listen to the answer, but also consider the source.*

This will give you some clues about where your self-image comes from. Families, especially, can help or hinder us in our efforts at self-improvement. Some family members and even people you think of as friends may have a stake in your being less than your best self. If you tune in to the message behind the words, you may also be able to identify those who will be valuable supporters of your weight-loss campaign and those whom you should steer clear of.

Use your reality check conversations with others to line up your cheering squad.

Make a page in your notebook called "Friends of My Diet," or whatever wording you like. List them by name and phone number and/or e-mail address. Make another list of people to avoid. Tell those you know you can count on that you want to lose weight and become more fit. Ask them to be helpful and tell them how they can support you.

How others can support you

There are many simple and easy ways people can lend you support. Here are some examples. They can:

a) Join you for a walk, jog, bike ride, or other active exercise

b) Keep your weight-loss goals in mind when planning social meals to which you are invited

c) Be honest, but not cruel, about how you look, especially when you start looking better

d) Be available, by phone or in person, when you need extra motivation or support

e) If appropriate, join you in a diet that will work for you both

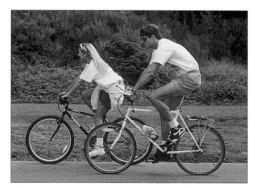

■ **If you are** *trying to build up your fitness program with a sport like cycling, get a friend to come with you and encourage you to go farther.*

f Help you not to break the rules that you've made for yourself, not even for a special occasion

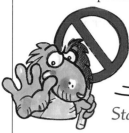

One of the best instructors in my gym ends every exercise class with a cool-down and round of deep breathing, during which she always tells us to eat lots of fruits and vegetables, drink lots of water, and exclude unsupportive people from our plans.

Stay away from negative people — you know who they are!

A simple summary

Make an accurate and honest assessment of whether and how much you are overweight before you begin any weight-loss plan.

Enlist your doctor or other health care professional in your plan to lose weight and become more active.

If you are severely overweight or obese (BMI 30 or greater), do not attempt to lose weight or increase your activity level without talking to a doctor first.

If you have a chronic disease or other serious health condition, do not attempt to lose weight or increase your activity level without talking to a doctor first.

If your BMI says your weight is normal, but you still think you're too fat, discuss your perception with your doctor before attempting to lose weight.

Spend an evening in front of the mirror (remembering to note your good points along with the bad) to help motivate you to lose weight and get fit.

Ask your friends and family to support you in your efforts to lose weight and become more active.

Exclude negative and unsupportive people from any discussions about your new lifestyle plan.

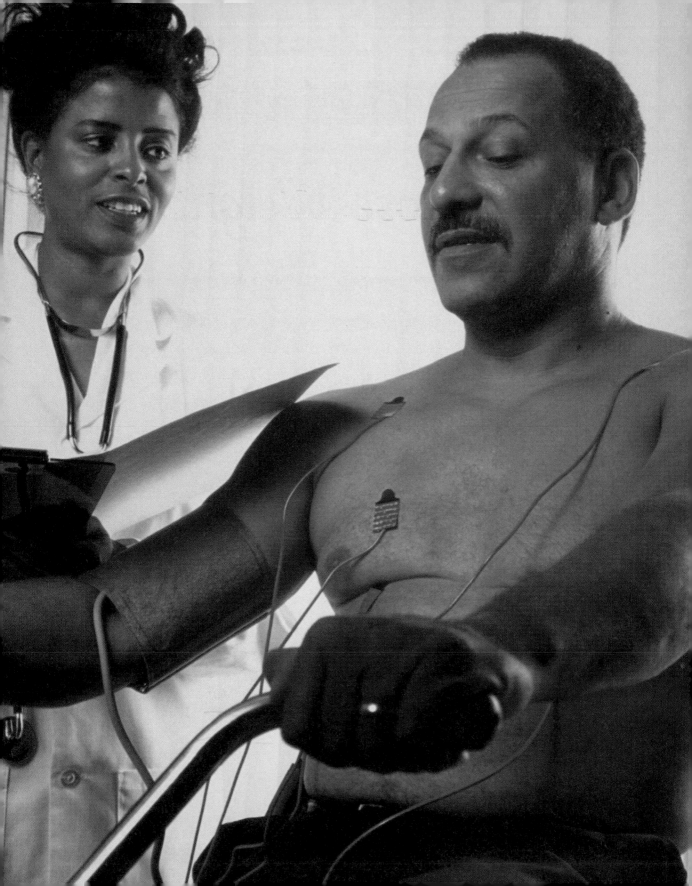

Chapter 2

Why Lose Weight?

Y OU PROBABLY PICKED UP THIS BOOK because you want to lose weight as a way of looking better. But the simple fact is, your weight is more than a matter of taste or aesthetics. It's a matter of health. I encourage you to read this chapter because it is, quite literally, the heart of the matter. Many of the problems associated with overweight affect your heart, and because of that, they affect your life. In this chapter, we discover why it is unhealthy to carry around excess weight.

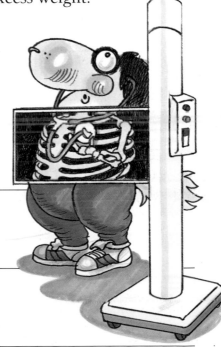

In this chapter...

✓ The medical perils of being overweight

✓ The health benefits of weight loss

✓ Other problems associated with overweight

LOSING EXCESS POUNDS WILL BE OF GREAT BENEFIT TO YOUR HEALTH

The medical perils of being overweight

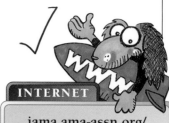

BEING OVERWEIGHT *increases your risk for many serious medical problems. The vast majority of overweight people suffer from one or more of the following conditions: diabetes, high cholesterol, high blood pressure, coronary artery disease, gall bladder disease, and arthritis. If that isn't bad enough, obesity is the second most important factor contributing to death in the United States. (It should come as no surprise that smoking is the first.)*

INTERNET

jama.ama-assn.org/ issues/v282n16

Articles in the American Medical Association's journal are written in language lay people may find difficult to understand. If you want to eavesdrop on doctors talking to each other, you'll find an issue of the journal devoted to the problems of being overweight at this address.

Diabetes

DEFINITION

Insulin is a hormone that converts sugar, starches, and other foods to energy. There are two main types of diabetes. Type 1 is the rarer of the two (representing only about five percent of all cases.) Sometimes called juvenile diabetes, type 1 is an autoimmune disease with strong genetic links. Far more common is type 2 diabetes, *which usually strikes people over age 45. Among the principal risk factors for type 2 diabetes are overweight, lack of regular exercise, and high cholesterol.*

Nearly 16 million Americans have diabetes, a metabolic disorder in which the body does not make enough *insulin* or cannot use it effectively. About 95 percent of people with diabetes have *type 2 diabetes*, which is closely tied to being overweight. Each year, more than 190,000 people die from diabetes or its many complications. For people who live with diabetes, it is a frequently disabling disease.

■ Diabetes is the leading cause of blindness in people between 20 and 74 years of age.

■ It is a major cause of kidney disease, requiring dialysis or kidney transplant.

■ People with diabetes are as much as four times more likely than others to have heart disease or suffer a stroke.

■ Diabetes causes nerve damage, which may require amputation of a toe, foot, or lower leg.

■ In men, diabetes is a frequent cause of erectile dysfunction.

There is no cure for diabetes, and it requires lifelong management and medication. All diabetics require a controlled diet to regulate blood sugar levels, and regular checkups to detect damage to the eyes, nerves, and blood vessels. There are ways to lower the risk of developing it, however. Although type 2 diabetes tends to run in families, people who are overweight and inactive are at much greater risk of contracting the disease.

Losing weight, controlling blood cholesterol levels, and engaging in some form of regular exercise are the best ways to prevent or delay the onset of type 2 diabetes.

INTERNET

diabetes.org

Check out the web site of the American Diabetes Association for general information, a test to determine your own risk for developing this disease, and tips and information on exercise, nutrition, and other ways to prevent, treat, and live with diabetes.

Cardiovascular disease

Cardiovascular disease (CVD) is an umbrella term covering disorders of the heart and blood vessels. It includes coronary artery disease, atherosclerosis, and hypertension (high blood pressure). Overweight, lack of exercise, stress, and a high-fat diet are major contributing factors to all CVD.

Coronary artery disease: In order to supply the rest of the body with blood, the heart muscle needs oxygenated blood itself. It gets it from the coronary arteries located on the outside wall of the heart. When one or more of these arteries are narrowed, blood flow is restricted or may be halted altogether. The result is coronary artery disease, the major underlying cause of heart attack.

One sign that the heart muscle is not getting enough oxygen are the chest pains of angina. This type of chest pain usually occurs during activity and is relieved by rest.

Atherosclerosis: This is a condition in which fatty deposits build up on the inside of arterial walls. As the arteries narrow, they cannot carry sufficient blood to the tissues. To compensate, the heart pumps harder, blood pressure increases, and many parts of the body are damaged as a result. Everything from poor circulation in the limbs to heart attack and stroke can be blamed on atherosclerosis.

Some people are more prone to atherosclerosis than others, but there is no question that a high-fat diet is a major contributor. People who are overweight, lead a sedentary lifestyle, and have high cholesterol levels are at much increased risk for developing atherosclerosis.

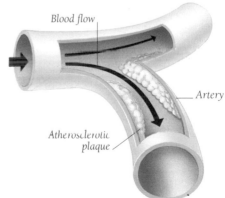

Blood flow

Artery

Atherosclerotic plaque

■ **Atherosclerosis** *occurs when fatty deposits build up on the insides of the artery walls, blocking the flow of blood.*

High blood pressure: Also called hypertension, high blood pressure is a condition in which the pressure exerted by blood as it is pumped through the arteries is consistently higher than normal. Normally, blood pressure at rest should not be greater than 120/80. Blood pressure is considered high if it is repeatedly and persistently higher than 140/90.

High blood pressure can damage the arteries, heart, and other organs, including the kidneys and the eyes. It increases the risk for heart attack, coronary artery disease, a *stroke*, kidney failure, and loss of sight due to damage to the retina. Hypertension is more common in men than women, and the incidence increases with age.

Being overweight is one of the most important risk factors for high blood pressure. People who are 20 percent overweight are eight times more likely to have high blood pressure than people of normal weight.

When your blood pressure is taken, the compression cuff on your arm causes a column of mercury to rise in a metered column. Two measurements are taken: the systolic reading is blood pressure at its highest, when the heart muscle contracts; the diastolic reading is blood pressure at its low point, when the heart muscle relaxes. In a blood pressure reading of 120/80, for example, the higher number (120) is systolic, the lower (80) is diastolic.

High blood cholesterol

Cholesterol is a fatty substance produced by the liver and present in some foods. In normal amounts, it is essential for many body processes, including producing hormones. Having "high cholesterol" is not always caused by eating foods high in cholesterol, but there is no question that a diet full of fatty foods is a contributing factor. Genetics play a role, which is why "cholesterol problems" often run in families. Lack of exercise, smoking, and being overweight must take a lot of the blame, however. There is also a connection between high cholesterol levels and diabetes.

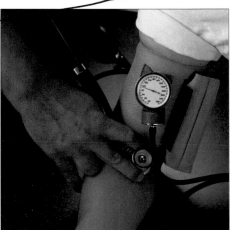

■ **When your blood** *pressure is taken, a compression cuff on your arm is pumped up and released to take two readings: systolic and diastolic.*

REDUCING STROKE RISK

A study published in the *Journal of the American Medical Association* found that people whose diets include lots of fruits and vegetables are less likely to suffer a stroke. According to the study, the best risk reducers are broccoli, cabbage, cauliflower, brussels sprouts, spinach, and citrus fruits.

ORANGE

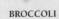

BROCCOLI

There are two important types of cholesterol: high-density lipoprotein (HDL) and low-density lipoprotein (LDL). To keep it simple, HDL is "good" cholesterol, because it protects against atherosclerosis. LDL is "bad" cholesterol, because it leaves deposits on the artery walls. So it's a good thing to have high HDL and low LDL.

Triglyceride is another fatty substance found in the blood as well as in some foods. Like LDL, high triglyceride levels are considered a bad thing. When the level of LDL and triglyceride in the blood is too high, the excess tends to be deposited on the inner walls of blood vessels. This narrows them, eventually resulting in atherosclerosis.

Cholesterol levels are measured by taking a sample of your blood, sometimes after you have not eaten for 12 hours or more. The results are usually reported as the total cholesterol level. Sometimes the levels of LDL, HDL, and triglycerides are also given separately, and a ratio of HDL to LDL is calculated.

A total cholesterol level above 200 is considered high. Among the risks associated with high blood cholesterol are high blood pressure, coronary artery disease, and stroke.

Being overweight and having high cholesterol levels is another one of those vicious circles. According to the experts, every 10 percent increase in weight increases cholesterol by 12 points. The more fat you consume, the more weight you gain; the more overweight you are, the higher your cholesterol. Exercise is the way to break out of the circle. Exercise burns calories, helping you use the food you eat as energy rather than store it as fat. It also lowers cholesterol levels.

Morbid obesity

This is overweight so extreme that it interferes with normal activities and body functions, including breathing. The complications of morbid *obesity* include diabetes and cardiovascular disease. In addition, sudden death is more common among people who are morbidly obese. They are also more prone to accidents and complications from surgery. Some cancers appear to be more common in people who are obese.

Obesity is classified as:

- **Mild:** 20–40 percent overweight

- **Moderate:** 40–100 percent overweight

- **Severe:** more than 100 percent overweight.

More recently, obesity has been defined in terms of body mass index (BMI). The World Health Organization classifies obesity as follows:

- **Class 1:** 30–34.9 BMI

- **Class 2:** 35–39.9 BMI

- **Class 3:** more than 40 BMI

DEFINITION

Obesity *has been defined as weight in excess of 20 percent of the standard for height, age, and gender.*

Strokes are twice as likely to occur in people who are obese

Obesity can cause breathlessness during exertion

The increase in mortality among people who are obese is due mainly to circulatory diseases

Seriously overweight people often have high cholesterol levels and can suffer from gallstones

People who are obese are vulnerable to skin chafing and fungal infections where folds of skin rub together, for example in the groin area

Extra weight can place strain on the joints in the legs

- **People who suffer** *from morbid obesity face many health problems, including back pain caused by excess body weight on the lower spine.*

EXERCISE AND BREAST CANCER RISK

According to a recent study, moderate to vigorous activity can decrease a woman's risk of breast cancer. An hour's exercise a day, seven days a week, decreased risk by 20 percent, but women who exercised for even a half hour daily were less likely to develop breast cancer than those who did not exercise at all. Walking, jogging, swimming, calisthenics, and rowing are among the choices suggested.

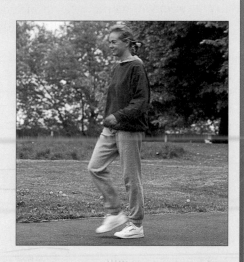

■ **Brisk walking,** *for at least a half hour daily, can keep you fit. It works all the body muscles, including the heart, and can give you protection from disease.*

Cancer

Even though cancer has many causes, some known and others unknown, certain cancers are known to be more prevalent in people who are overweight.

Although a direct causative link has not been established, being overweight has been implicated in cancers of the breast, uterus, prostate, and colon.

The American Cancer Society recommends limiting high-fat foods and eating lots of fruits, vegetables, grains, and beans. It also joins the chorus of those urging 30 minutes or more of exercise every day, and maintaining a healthy weight.

INTERNET

cancer.org

The American Cancer Society offers guidelines for diet and nutrition to help prevent cancer.

Other health risks

Lung problems: Excess fat, especially on the trunk, exerts pressure on the diaphragm and interferes with normal breathing. It is not unusual for people who are overweight to suffer from shortness of breath. Not only do they have problems getting enough oxygen, they also have problems exhaling carbon dioxide. This can make them feel sleepy even when they are getting plenty of sleep.

Obese people who often feel sleepy and short of breath find it very difficult to be physically active – a vicious circle.

Gall bladder disease: The gall bladder is a small, saclike organ that stores gall, which is manufactured by the liver and is used to break down food molecules. It can become clogged with gallstones, which consist mainly of cholesterol. Pain, inflammation, and infection frequently result. Sometimes the infection spreads, causing serious complications.

People who are overweight or have a high-fat diet are at greatest risk of developing gallstones and gall bladder disease.

Joint diseases: Osteoarthritis and gout are two painful and debilitating joint disorders that are often related to overweight. Osteoarthritis is common in women over 60, though men suffer from it as well. It is a "wear-and-tear" condition that results

THE OVERWEIGHT SMOKER

If you had to choose between smoking and overweight as the greater threat to your health, smoking would certainly win. But what do you do if you are living with both? Smoking is a villain in most of the medical problems associated with overweight: heart and lung problems, diabetes and cancer, not to mention poor circulation, osteoporosis, and a host of other ailments. Overweight smokers are hit with a double whammy.

Overweight smokers often cling to their habit because they believe they will gain even more weight if they quit. It is true that people tend to gain some weight during the early period of kicking the habit. Temporary metabolic changes may be responsible, but more likely food is being used for oral gratification in the absence of a cigarette.

Still, quitting smoking and losing weight are the two most important lifesaving efforts a person can make. Because of their special difficulties, overweight smokers should work with a doctor as they may need behavioral therapy and drug assistance.

■ **Smoking cigarettes** *is very damaging to health and highly dangerous for those who are overweight. Quitting will often need a doctor's assistance.*

OVERWEIGHT CHILDREN AND TEENS

Being overweight has reached epidemic proportions in the youngest generation. Since 1980, the rate of childhood obesity has nearly doubled. One out of five American teenagers is seriously overweight. Poor eating habits and being glued to the television or computer screen have been cited as contributing to the sorry state of our nation's youth.

The health implications are very serious indeed. More than half of all overweight children between the ages of 5 and 10 already have one or more of the health

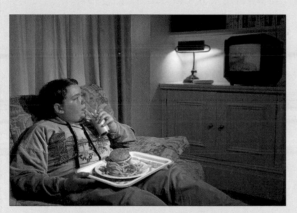

problems we've been talking about: high cholesterol, high blood pressure, or metabolic abnormalities that eventually lead to diabetes. Overweight children grow up to be overweight, and often obese, adults.

■ **An obsession with** *junk food, TV, and the Internet is creating a nation of overweight children. Many children exercise little and suffer from health problems.*

when the cartilage that protects the ends of joints deteriorates. The joints most commonly affected are the hips and knees, which bear most of our weight. It should come as no surprise, therefore, that people who bear a lot of weight tend to suffer more often, earlier in life, and more severely from arthritis.

Trivia...

Are people who are overweight more likely to snore? Yes. That's because fatty tissue at the back of their throat obstructs breathing passages when they are lying down.

If arthritis is more common in women, men are the ones who suffer more often from gout. This painful inflammation of the joints often strikes the big toe. It is associated with overweight and excessive alcohol use. Kidney complications are sometimes seen in people who have both gout and diabetes.

Although these joint diseases can be treated with drugs that relieve pain and inflammation and help avoid further destruction of bone and tissue, lifestyle changes may also help. Weight loss is strongly recommended for overweight joint-disease patients.

How's Your Health?

Ideally, you see a doctor regularly so your health is closely monitored. Nonetheless, you are the guardian of your own health, and in this managed-care world it is more important than ever that you protect your own health interests.

The following self-quiz is a simple way for you to see, in black and white, if you have any health problems that can be attributed to being overweight and lack of fitness or that would benefit from weight loss and regular exercise. Write the answers in the spaces provided in this book or make a photocopy for your personal database and take it with you to your next doctor's appointment.

This quiz will help you and your doctor become health-care and weight-loss partners. It may also provide important motivation to help you reach your weight-loss goals.

Diabetes risk

		Yes	No
1	Have you been diagnosed with diabetes?	☐	☑
2	Have you ever had an abnormally high blood sugar test result?	☐	☑
3	If so, were you advised to have another test at some point in the future?	☐	☑
4	Did you follow that advice?	☐	☑

Cardiovascular disease risk

		Yes	No
5	Have you ever been told you have abnormally high blood pressure (hypertension)?	☑	☐
6	If so, did you receive medical advice related to this health problem?	☑	☐
7	Was medication prescribed for it?	☐	☑
8	Have you followed the advice and/or taken the medication?	☑	☐

9 Have you ever been diagnosed with heart disease
   or any other heart condition? ☐ ☑

10 Have you ever experienced chest pain during exercise? ☐ ☑

11 If so, have you reported this to a doctor? ☐ ☑

12 If you have reported it, what were you told? ☐̶̶̶̶̶☐

High blood cholesterol risk

		YES	NO
13	Have you ever had a test for blood cholesterol?	☑	☐
14	Do you remember the result?	☑	☐

15 If so, what was it? _____ oK _____

16	Were you told that it was abnormally high?	☐	☑
17	If so, was cholesterol-lowering medication prescribed for you?	☐	☑
18	Are you still taking it?	☐̶̶̶	☑̶

Other health risks

		YES	NO
19	Have you ever been diagnosed with cancer of the breast, colon, or prostate?	☐	☑
20	Do you have arthritis or periodic or constant pain in one or more weight-bearing joints such as your hips, knees, or ankles?	☐	☑
21	Do you have pain in one or both big toes?	☐	☑
22	Have you ever had gallstones or a gall bladder attack?	☑	☐
23	Has anyone ever told you that you snore or frequently awaken with a loud snort in the middle of sleeping?	☑	☐
24	Do you feel breathless when climbing a few stairs or walking a short distance?	☑	☐

Your family history

Even if you are satisfied with your weight, there may be health reasons why you should keep it under control. Knowing your family history will provide clues to what the future may hold if you do not add sensible eating and regular physical activity to your lifestyle.

		YES	NO
25	Does overweight run in your family?	✓	☐
26	Did any member of your family develop diabetes in adulthood?	✓	☐
27	Has any member of your family been told he or she has high cholesterol?	✓	☐
28	Has any member of your family been diagnosed with high blood pressure (hypertension)?	✓	☐
29	Does any member of your family have heart disease?	✓	☐
30	Has any member of your family suffered or died from a heart attack?	✓	☐
31	Has any member of your family suffered or died from a stroke?	☐	✓
32	Has any member of your family suffered or died from cancer of the breast, colon, or prostate?	✓	☐

NOTES

_____

_____

_____

_____

_____

_____

The health benefits of weight loss ✓

30 min *walk* ✱

AFTER ALL THIS GLOOM AND DOOM, *you're probably ready for some good news. If being overweight is bad for your health (and it is), then losing weight is the best cure.*

According to the experts, a weight loss of as little as 5 to 10 percent reduces an obese adult's risk of developing type 2 diabetes, high blood pressure, high cholesterol, and arthritis. Overweight people already suffering from these conditions usually improve when they lose weight. Losing weight also reduces the incidence of a whole host of heart and lung disorders.

If you're wondering why you should lose weight, I can't think of a better answer.

Trivia... ✓
You may be able to walk your way to a healthy heart. A study of elderly men aged 61 to 81 showed that those who walked more than 1½ miles a day had half the risk of coronary heart disease of men who walked less than a quarter mile a day.

Other problems associated with overweight

EVEN THOUGH HEALTH CONSIDERATIONS *are probably the strongest argument in favor of losing weight, being overweight can make your life difficult in many other ways. If staying healthy and preventing disease do not motivate you, maybe the aesthetic, social, emotional, and financial consequences of being overweight will give you the push you need.*

Aesthetic

Especially in our society, overweight is not the "look we like." The most attractive clothing is designed for slimmer folks. Even if you have given up on dressing in the latest fashion, it is hard to look your best when your clothes are either too tight or utterly shapeless to hide your form.

Social

Not looking your best has social consequences as well. First impressions count for a lot, and, like it or not, first impressions are usually visual ones. Whether you're hoping for a date, a friend, a job offer, or just not to be the last one chosen for the Saturday softball game, you're at a disadvantage if you're overweight. It may feel unfair, and it probably is, but that's the way it's been since grade school and the way it is now.

Plain and simple, there are strong social biases against fatties. Many people regard being overweight as a character flaw, a sign of slovenliness and lack of self-control.

Emotional

Many of the negative responses of others are shared by heavy people themselves. Self-esteem and a positive self-image are harder to come by when you are overweight. Depression often accompanies weight problems, sometimes as cause and sometimes as a result. People who are depressed tend also to be physically inactive. It's another one of those vicious circles.

Being more active can help lift depression just as it helps you lose weight. Many of the body chemicals that influence mood are influenced in turn by physical exertion.

Financial

Obesity makes a dent in the American economy of more than $100 billion every year, including the cost of health care and productivity that is lost to death and disability from weight-related causes.

■ **Doing some regular** *exercise can help boost your confidence when you are trying to lose weight. Exerting your body encourages the release of endorphins, or "happy hormones," making you feel good about yourself.*

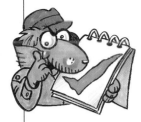

On an individual level, people who are overweight spend more money on medical care than people of normal weight.

Overweight people suffer from higher rates of disease and more complications. They also are involved in more accidents that result in injury. They are hospitalized more often and tend to suffer more complications from surgery and other medical procedures. People who are overweight may also experience more difficulty in getting life insurance because of their high-risk status. Those who are able to get insurance will often pay higher premiums.

All of this costs money. So if saving your life is not enough to make you lose weight, maybe saving your money is!

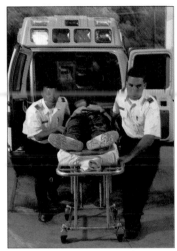

■ **If you are overweight** *you are more likely to have health complications that require treatment in hospital and suffer injuries from accidents. Recovery rates are also likely to be slower.*

A simple summary

✓ Being overweight increases the risk for many serious medical problems, including diabetes, heart and lung diseases, cancer, gall bladder disease, and arthritis.

✓ Discussing the health risks of overweight with your doctor can be a powerful weight-loss motivator.

✓ The high incidence of being overweight among children and teens is of particular concern for our nation's future health.

✓ Being overweight has many negative aesthetic, social, emotional, and financial consequences.

✓ Losing weight has immediate and measurable health benefits. It is one of the most effective preventive health strategies you can take.

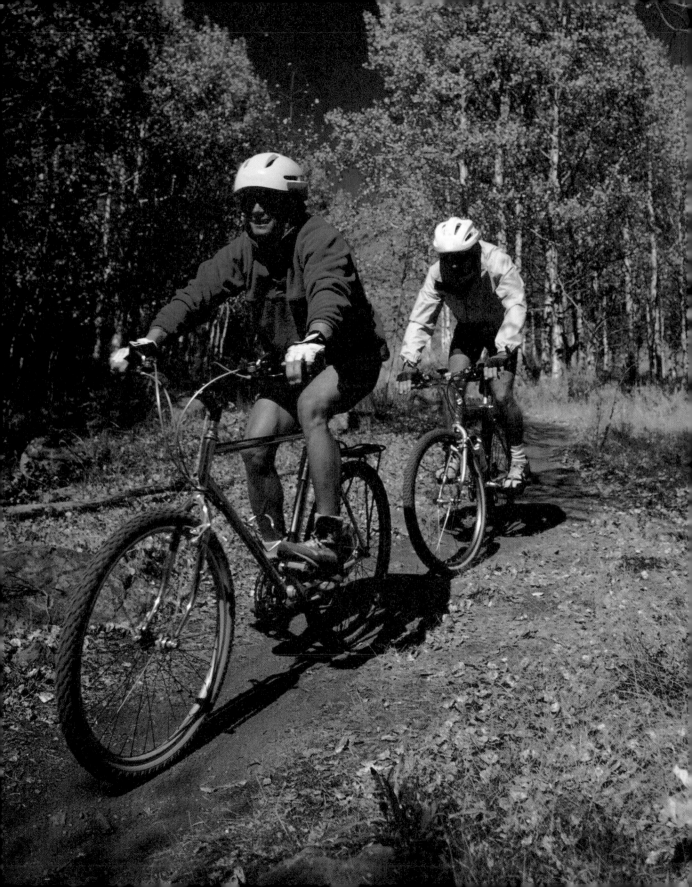

Chapter 3

Fitness Is the Goal

THE MOST SENSIBLE WAY to think about weight loss is as part of an overall effort to get and stay fit. In this chapter, we'll look at the components of fitness and why they are important to overall health. We'll consider the roles that the heart and other muscles play in fitness. Making the choice to lose weight is an important part of choosing to get fit.

In this chapter...

✓ What is fitness?

✓ Your heart is the most important muscle in your body

✓ What about all those other muscles?

✓ Fitness for all

✓ Fitness is a lifestyle choice

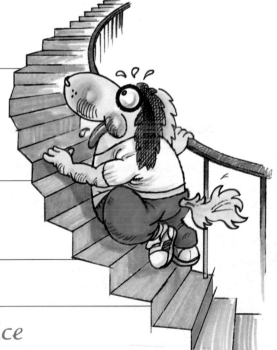

IMPROVED STRENGTH, ENDURANCE, AND FLEXIBILITY ARE AMONG THE BENEFITS OF AN ACTIVE LIFESTYLE

What is fitness?

Cardiovascular *is an umbrella word that covers the heart and blood vessels. There are two kinds of blood vessels: the arteries, which carry oxygen-rich blood from the heart, and the veins, which return with oxygen-depleted blood.*
The term **cardiorespiratory** *refers to the heart and lungs working together to pump oxygenated blood.*
Aerobic *means "in the presence of oxygen." Aerobic exercise is any sustained physical activity, such as jogging, running, swimming, or aerobic dancing, that increases the supply of oxygen, and therefore energy, to the muscles.*

TO KEEP IT SIMPLE, *physical fitness is the ability of your body to do the work required of it. Although all body systems contribute to fitness, the muscles are the primary actors. In order to do their work, muscles need oxygen. They get it from blood, which is oxygenated by the lungs and pumped by the heart. Fitness depends on healthy lungs and a healthy heart supplying plenty of oxygen to strong muscles.*

The components of fitness

There are three main components of physical fitness, all of which are related.

Endurance: Also called *cardiovascular*, *cardiorespiratory*, or *aerobic* fitness, endurance depends on the heart, lungs, and blood vessels delivering oxygen-rich blood efficiently to all tissues in the body, including the muscles, and carrying away carbon dioxide and other waste products. To put it simply, aerobic fitness = endurance. Aerobic exercise increases your endurance.

Feeling out of breath is a sign that you've come to the end of your aerobic endurance.

Strength: This is the ability of your muscles to exert force to push, pull, or lift an object, including your own body. To put it simply, muscular fitness = strength + endurance.

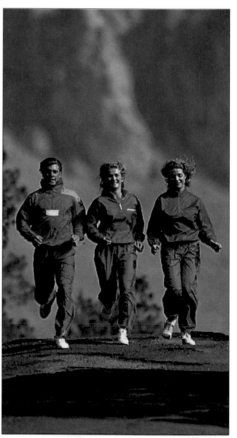

■ **Aerobic exercise** *such as running works the lungs and heart hard. It is an important part of a physical fitness regime.*

The number of times you can lift a given weight (or the number of exercise reps you can do, in weight-training lingo) is a good way to measure your muscular fitness.

Strength training with light weights increases your muscular fitness, as you'll see later in this chapter.

Flexibility: Also referred to as range of motion, flexibility is the ability to bend and stretch easily. Muscles, joints, and the tissues that connect them (ligaments and tendons) all play a major part in how well you can bend and stretch.

Feeling stiff when you try to touch your toes is a sign that you lack flexibility. Stretching exercises increase your flexibility.

■ **Stretching** *helps you maintain flexibility and suppleness in your muscles. An exercise class is a good place to learn how to do stretching exercises properly.*

HOW FIT ARE WE AS A NATION?

Not very, as it turns out. The Department of Health and Human Services set specific targets for physical activity and fitness as part of an overall effort to improve public health called Healthy People 2000. When they looked at the results at the end of 1999, they found that we fell short of many of the intended goals.

1 Goal: Light to moderate physical activity for at least 30 minutes, 5 or more times per week.

Target: 30 percent of the population aged 18 and older.

Reality: Less than 25 percent.

2 Goal: Vigorous physical activity for at least 20 minutes, 3 or more days a week.

Target: 20 percent of the population aged 18 and older.

Reality: 16 percent.

Target: 75 percent of students in grades 9–12.

Reality: 64 percent.

And here's some more bad news:

a The goal was to reduce the percentage of the total population aged 18 and older who engage in no leisure-time physical activity to 15 percent; the reality was 24 percent.

b The proportion of adolescents in grades 9 to 12 who participate in daily school physical education decreased from 42 percent in 1991 to 27 percent in 1999. The Healthy People 2000 target was 50 percent.

c Obesity and low levels of physical activity account for the large percentage of recruits who fail to complete military basic training.

New fitness goals have been set for the year 2010. Will America measure up by then? Will you?

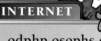

INTERNET

odphp.osophs.dhhs. gov/pubs/hp2000/

If you want to know more about national fitness goals, check out the Healthy People 2000 web site. You'll also find the year 2010 targets – our fitness benchmarks for the new millennium.

Your heart is the most important muscle in your body

IT'S ABOUT THE SIZE OF YOUR FIST, but your heart is the powerhouse of the cardiovascular system. It can pump more than a gallon of blood around your body every minute, 60 minutes an hour, 24 hours a day. That comes to more than 1,400 round trips!

Traveling through the arteries, the blood carries essential nutrients and oxygen to the farthest reaches of your body. After returning to the heart through the veins, the blood is then pumped to the lungs, where carbon dioxide and other waste gases are removed and oxygen is replenished.

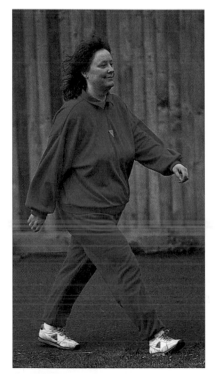

■ **Starting an exercise** *program is hard for people who are overweight. Walking is ideal; start with short distances and slowly increase them.*

All the while, your heart is doing the work. This process goes on when you are awake and when you are asleep. And you couldn't live without it.

Your heart during exercise

If the normal speed of circulation is about 10.5 pints per minute, the rate during exercise is much greater than that. Not only is blood pumped at a faster rate, but its destination is altered during exercise. More blood is routed to the muscles – as much as 12 times the normal volume – and away from the digestive system, which may be visited by a third less blood than usual during this time.

The overweight heart

You already know about the health risks of being overweight. Many of them have to do with the heart. The simple fact is that being overweight and inactive has wide-ranging negative effects on the entire cardiovascular system.

In addition, people who are overweight tend to have less endurance, so it is difficult for them to engage in sustained physical activity. It is a vicious circle, since being active would help them become more fit, but their very lack of fitness is preventing them from being active. The best way out of the vicious circle is to start slowly, with a small amount of low-intensity exercise. Walking is a good choice. Gentle stretching is another.

If you are extremely overweight or have or suspect you have heart problems, do not begin any sort of exercise program, no matter how modest, until you have talked to your doctor about it.

What about all those other muscles?

IF THE HEART *is the most important muscle for endurance, then strength and flexibility are the territory of your skeletal muscles. These are the muscles that make it possible for us to move, lift things, and even to stand up. Muscles also give shape to the body. Without muscles, we'd be little more than a bag of bones.*

The way to increase muscular strength is make muscles do the work they were designed to do. Working against resistance – pushing or lifting – gives muscles their tone. The more you do it, the stronger you become. Within limits.

Hormones, particularly the hormone testosterone, play a part in muscle development. The more testosterone you have, the more you'll be able to strengthen and build up your muscles. Although women produce some testosterone, men produce a lot more. That's why men look more muscular than women and why working out produces a more sculptured look in men.

Before puberty, testosterone is in short supply in both sexes, so preteens should be discouraged from "pumping iron."

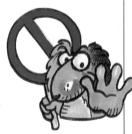

Preteens should not work out. It won't give them bulging muscles, but it may damage growing bones and connective tissues.

Developing, strengthening, and toning

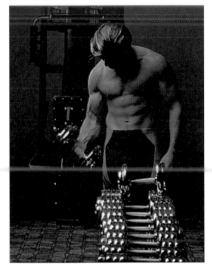

■ **Training** *with heavy weights is used to develop bulky muscles: lighter weights are used to improve strength.*

Speaking of bulging muscles, this is a good time to point out the difference between weight training and strength training. Weight training involves lifting increasingly heavy weights with the aim of developing bulging muscles. In strength training, you lift light weights (typically 1 to 3 pounds and never more than 10 pounds) repeatedly (usually in sets of 10 to 12 repetitions, or reps) until the muscles tire. The result is stronger and more toned muscles, not necessarily larger ones.

Strength training with weights is one way to build strength and condition muscles, but it is not the only way. Running, jumping, swimming, climbing stairs, playing sports are all muscle builders. True fitness – endurance, strength, and flexibility – does not require huge muscles. In fact, the muscle-bound look may limit your flexibility.

When all is said and done, the best way to strengthen muscles is to use them.

Muscles as a sign of fitness

The payoff of working your muscles is more than increased strength. Strength training increases metabolism, the process by which the body turns food into energy. You'll be learning more about metabolism in Chapter 5, but for now just remember this piece of good news: The faster your metabolism, the more fat you burn, making it easier to keep your weight under control.

Since it takes more energy to maintain muscles than fat, the greater your muscle mass, the more calories you burn every time you move a muscle.

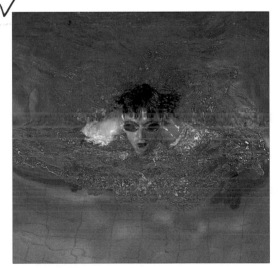

■ **Swimming is a** *great sport for all ages. It's ideal for strengthening muscles without straining them because water supports the body, and it's good aerobic exercise, too.*

Steroids and Other Muscle-Building Supplements

Athletes who use anabolic steroids and other synthetic muscle-building compounds have put the spotlight on a disturbing trend. Many people – most of them male, many of them young – have tried to build their bodies by taking these supplements. There is some question whether they are effective, but there is no question that they are dangerous. The worst thing is that many "muscle enhancers" are available without a prescription. Creatine, androstenedione, and dehydroepiandrosterone (DHEA) are the most popular, but there are others marketed under a variety of names. Anabolic steroids, which are synthetic versions of testosterone, require a doctor's prescription, but there are many underground sources of these very potent drugs.

A study of the hormone androstenedione found that it was no more effective than exercise alone in building muscles, despite the tempting example of home-run slugger Mark McGwire. It can cause acne, prostate enlargement in men, and a drop in levels of HDL (the "good" cholesterol). DHEA has similar side effects; in addition, women taking it may have increased facial hair and irregular or missed menstrual periods. Creatine can stress the kidneys and cause stomach problems.

Nutritional supplements are not required by law to be tested for safety and effectiveness as prescription drugs are. I'll talk more about this loophole and what it means to your health in later chapters. But for now, the simple truth is that whether they work or not, steroids and other muscle enhancers have been reported to cause the following problems:

- Heart damage
- Increased blood clotting that can lead to heart attack or stroke
- Increased levels of "bad" (LDL) and decreased levels of "good" (HDL) cholesterol
- Liver damage
- Diarrhea, nausea, and other digestive disturbances
- Changes in both male and female reproductive systems, including shrinkage of the testicles, reduced sperm count, and irregular menstruation
- Acne
- Hair loss or, in women, excess body hair
- Mood changes, including depression, irritability, and mood swings

Enough said?

Fitness for all

FITNESS IMPROVES HEALTH and quality of life for everyone, no matter your age or ability. It's as important for seniors as it is for children, as vital for people with physical disabilities or chronic illnesses as it is for those in shape.

It's prime time: fitness for adults

You are living the best years of your life. The growing pains of adolescence are over, and you are not yet subject to the infirmities of age. Now is the time to get up and get moving. Use the vigor of your middle years to develop habits you can keep for a lifetime.

Be sure to build some kind of activity into every day. It need not take a lot of time, but it may mean trading some less active pursuits for those that enhance fitness.

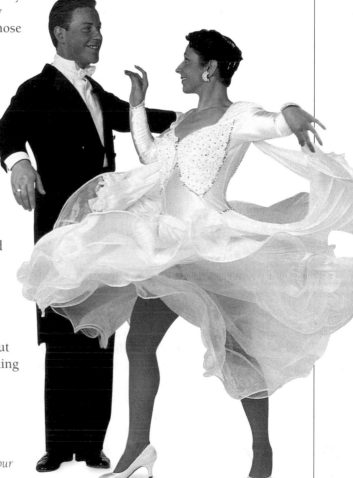

Your goal should be 30 minutes of activity a day, but if that seems hard to schedule, start with 15. Chances are you will quickly feel the benefits and want to do more, not less.

In Chapter 12, we'll be looking at the wide range of exercise options. The trick is to find something that suits your interests and feels like fun. You don't have to join a gym, but you might consider ballroom dancing. You don't have to take a morning run, but how about a lunchtime stroll? You don't have to buy fancy exercise equipment, but what about dusting off that bicycle in the garage and taking it for a spin? The possibilities are limitless.

■ **Choose an active** *pastime that you enjoy. Ballroom dancing can be sociable and great exercise, increasing your endurance, stamina, and flexibility.*

Make it a family affair

If you have children or teens, do them and yourself a favor by making fitness part of your family values.

According to Healthy People 2000, not a single state in the country mandates daily physical education in schools. The most recent figures show that less than one quarter of American high school students spend 30 minutes one or more times a week in gym class. Among elementary and secondary schools, fewer than 36 percent offer daily phys ed classes of any sort. Is it any wonder that young people are more overweight and less fit today than in previous generations?

Don't rely on schools to provide enough physical activity for your children.

Habits formed in childhood will last a lifetime: If you raise your children to be physically active, the chances are good that they will grow up to be active, and fit, adults. One of the best ways to ensure this is to be a good role model yourself. If you follow an active lifestyle and make fitness the goal, your children are more likely to do the same. On the other hand, it will be hard to sell them on fitness if they see you sitting around all day.

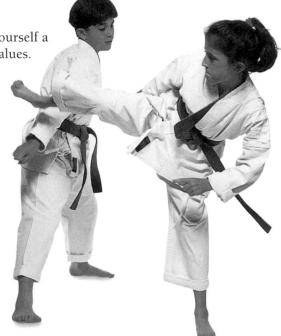

■ **Martial arts have** *great appeal for children and adults alike. Karate is a form of self-defense that involves punching, kicking, and blocking techniques. It helps cardiovascular fitness and increases muscle tone.*

INTERNET

drkoop.com /wellness/fitness

Former Surgeon General C. Everett Koop wants America to get fit. The Fitness Center area at drkoop.com offers information, inspiration, facts, and ideas to help you get started.

You're never too old

My mother is comfortably into her 80s. Every morning before breakfast, she does 20 minutes of stretching exercise. Before dinner she swims 10 laps. Twice a week she goes to an exercise or yoga class, and on off days she takes a brisk walk. She can touch her toes, climb a flight of stairs without panting, and she passes her annual physicals with flying colors. More important, though, she has all her marbles and a positive outlook on life. There is no question that her years-long habit of regular physical activity is responsible. But even older people who are not blessed with my mother's vigor and good health, or who did not get her head start on fitness, can make physical activity part of their daily lives.

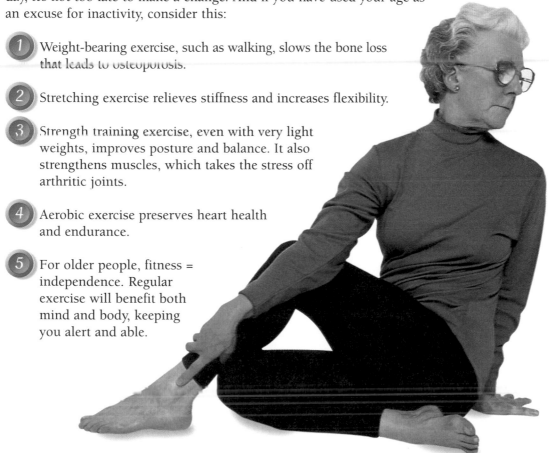

As we grow older, we naturally lose muscle mass. Hormonal and other age-related body changes mean the muscle-building days are over.

Don't stop exercising as you age, it's important to keep the muscles you have in good tone.

If you are an active older person, keep it up. If activity is not a regular part of your day, it's not too late to make a change. And if you have used your age as an excuse for inactivity, consider this:

1. Weight-bearing exercise, such as walking, slows the bone loss that leads to osteoporosis.

2. Stretching exercise relieves stiffness and increases flexibility.

3. Strength training exercise, even with very light weights, improves posture and balance. It also strengthens muscles, which takes the stress off arthritic joints.

4. Aerobic exercise preserves heart health and endurance.

5. For older people, fitness = independence. Regular exercise will benefit both mind and body, keeping you alert and able.

■ **In later life,** *doing regular stretching exercises can keep you supple and offset any stiffness that is starting to appear in your joints.*

Focus on the abled part

There is no question that among the challenges faced by people with physical disabilities is how they can be active and stay fit. It is not impossible, but it takes an extra effort and often assistance from others to find accessible and appropriate activities.

Depending on the disability, some parts of the body may be more able than others to lift, bend, stretch, and move. Achieving aerobic intensity may or may not be possible, but strengthening some muscle groups may be a reasonable aim. Maintaining good flexibility is another benefit worth striving for.

People with disabilities should talk with their doctor or other health-care provider about what they can and should be doing to stay fit. They may benefit from the help of a physical therapist, personal trainer, or special equipment, and they may be eligible for assistance in covering the cost.

Fitness is a lifestyle choice

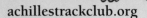

INTERNET

achillestrackclub.org

Achilles Track Club is a worldwide nonprofit organization that encourages people with all kinds of disabilities to enjoy the benefits of running and walking and to participate in short- and long-distance recreational and competitive running. To find out more, including the location of the local chapter nearest you, visit their web site.

DO YOU WANT TO KNOW the real weight-loss "secret"? It's not a special diet. It's not a supplement or pill. It's not a device or medical procedure. The real secret of achieving and maintaining a healthy weight is to get and stay fit. Without any doubt, you will find that an active lifestyle will help you lose weight. It will also keep you focused in a positive and energetic way that will make everything you do easier.

Leading an active life is a habit, just as being a sedentary stay-at-home is. And like any habit, you tend to do it without thinking or planning. It just comes naturally. And you miss it when you don't do it. But how wonderful to form a habit that is good for you.

The trick is simply to replace bad habits with good ones.

(a) If you spend the first hour of your day watching a morning news program while dunking a donut in your coffee, why not watch the news while stretching instead? Or don your headphones and listen to the news while you take a morning walk or run?

(b) If you take a midday break by snacking while phoning a friend, why not arrange to meet your friend and go for a walk instead?

c If your idea of "quality time" with your kids is to pick them up in the car after school, swing by the local fast food emporium, and then spend a few hours watching television with them, why not meet them with bikes or skates and take the long way home?

d If you spend your weekends at the mall, why not try going for a walk in the woods or spend a day at the gym instead?

Can you think of other habits you can change so they spell FIT instead of SIT?

■ **Take advantage of** *your free time on weekends to go out walking with family or friends. It's enjoyable and it will help to increase your fitness levels.*

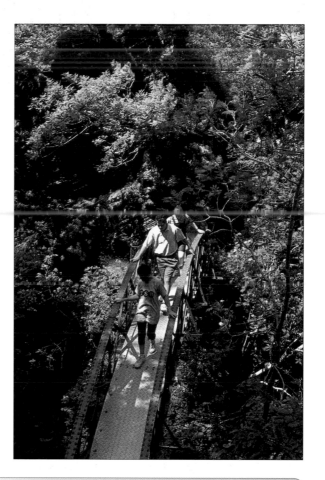

A simple summary

✔ Fitness is a combination of endurance, strength, and flexibility.

✔ A healthy heart is the keystone of fitness.

✔ Muscular strength and endurance are signs of fitness; muscular bulk is not.

✔ Being overweight makes your heart work too hard to be fit.

✔ A minimum of 30 minutes of physical activity should be part of your life every day.

✔ Fitness should be your goal throughout life. You are never too young or too old to be fit.

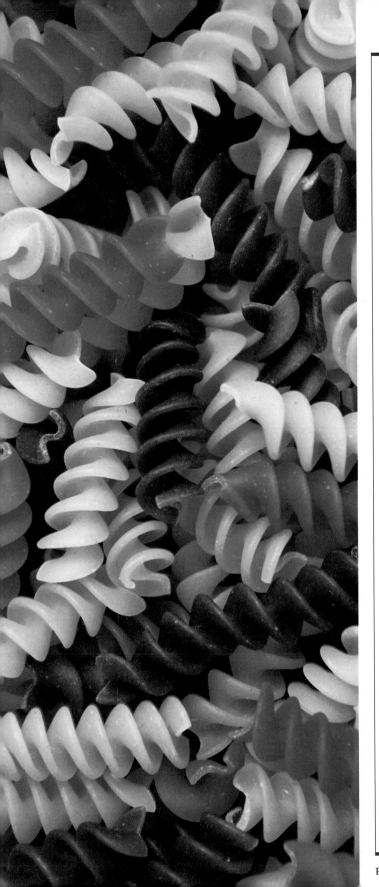

PART TWO

PASTA IS A GOOD SOURCE OF CARBOHYDRATES

LEARNING ABOUT IT

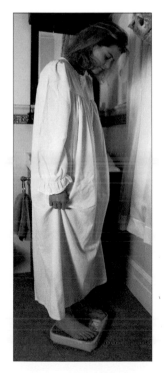

Y OU MAY THINK you know everything you need to know about *weight loss*. After all, there are a zillion books on the subject, and more magazine articles. You can't turn on the television or walk the supermarket aisles without being bombarded with information, and misinformation, on the subject.

How do you choose the weight-loss strategy that is right for you? The best way to begin is with a review of nutrition *facts*. This part of the book will help you separate the myths from the reality and prepare you to make the important choices that lie before you in your quest for permanent and *healthy* weight loss. So, get ready to learn everything there is to know about calories and carbohydrates, pounds and protein, vitamins and vitality. And the facts, not the fiction, about fat.

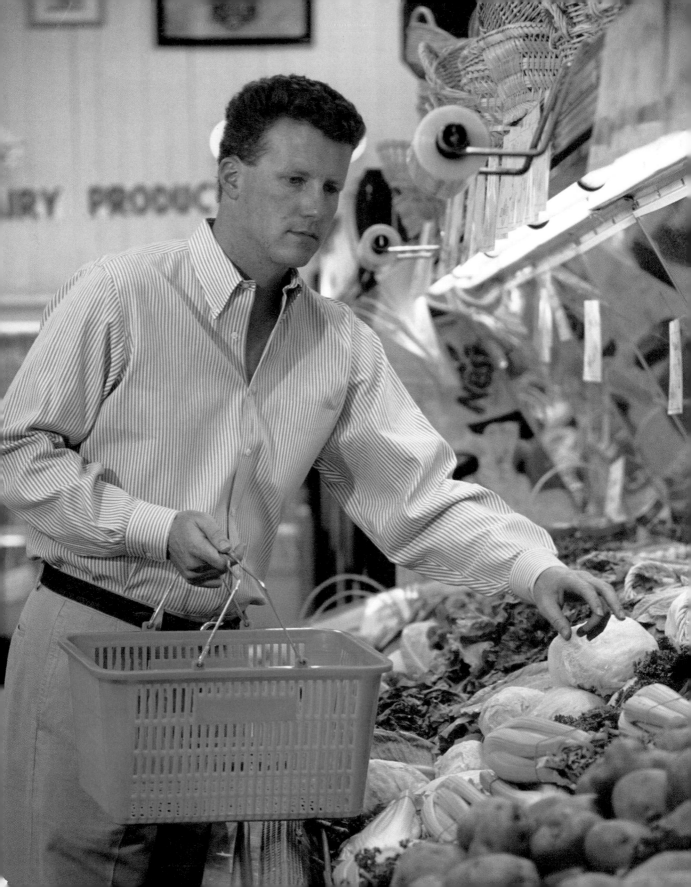

Chapter 4

The ABCs of Nutrition

THIS CHAPTER TAKES US BACK to elementary school health and nutrition class. You may think you know your ABCs, but many people seem to forget them when it comes to eating and losing weight, which is why they try diets that exclude one or more food groups or are unbalanced in other ways. We'll begin by looking at the major nutrient and micronutrient groups. We'll also examine what a balanced diet means and the tools you can use to design a healthful eating program.

In this chapter...

✓ Nutrition basics

✓ Body fuel

✓ Life's building blocks

✓ The skinny on fats

✓ The mighty micronutrients

✓ How to read a food label

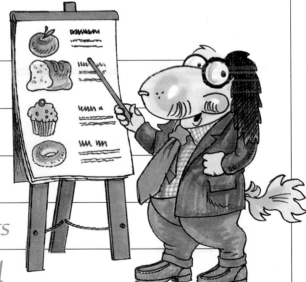

KNOWING WHAT CONSTITUTES A BALANCED DIET WILL HELP YOU MAKE THE RIGHT FOOD CHOICES

Nutrition basics

EVEN THOUGH WE'LL BE LOOKING at each group separately, most foods contain a combination of nutrients, though one or another might predominate. Rarely will you encounter a "pure" protein or carbohydrate, and even though pure fats are more common, most of the fat you eat comes along with carbohydrates and protein. This is even more true of vitamins and minerals, which occur naturally in or are added to many foods.

INTERNET

warp.nal.usda.gov:80/ fnic/dga

You can find the latest Dietary Guidelines for Americans at the U.S. Department of Agriculture's Food and Nutrition Information Center. There's lots of solid information about nutrition and useful links to other sites.

Nutrients are typically measured in metric units: grams for protein, carbohydrates and fats, and milligrams and micrograms for vitamins and minerals.

If you haven't "gone metric" yet, milligrams (mg) and micrograms (mcg) are teeny amounts; a gram (g) is equal to about 0.035 ounces; a kilogram (kg, or 1,000 grams) is equal to 2.2 pounds.

Even in the United States, nutrition labels on packaged foods will refer to grams of fat, protein, and carbohydrate.

Recommended daily amounts (RDA) of nutrients are for the "average" person. They do not take into account a specific individual's age, gender, weight, activity level, and health status. Think of these as guidelines only.

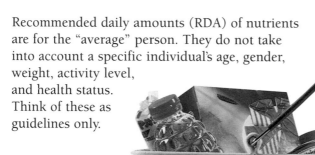

■ **Packaged food labels** *state which nutrients the product contains, how much of each nutrient is provided, plus the recommended daily amounts. Think of RDAs as guidelines only, since they won't specifically apply to you.*

Body fuel

CARBOHYDRATES ARE OUR *main source of energy. They provide most of the fuel your body uses to function. The brain relies exclusively on carbohydrates to do its work. Tell that to the diet meisters who want you to eliminate carbohydrates.*

There are several subtypes of carbohydrates:

1. Simple carbohydrates: Also known as sugars or saccharides. In addition to the kind of sugar you sprinkle on your cereal, simple carbohydrates are found in milk, fruits, and many vegetables. Sucrose, lactose, fructose, dextrose, and maltose are all simple carbohydrates. In the body they are converted to glucose, the technical name for blood sugar.

   Sugars are simple molecules, so your body breaks them down quickly. The "energy burst" or "sugar high" you get after eating sweets is evidence of this speedy conversion.

■ **If you sprinkle** *sugar on cereal, you're eating carbohydrate in its simplest form. This type of sugar gets into the bloodstream fast, giving you a quick blast of energy.*

■ **Fruits provide** *simple carbohydrates, most often in the form of fructose. They also contain plenty of fiber and water.*

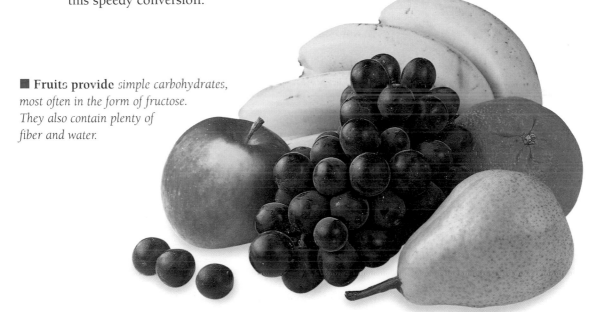

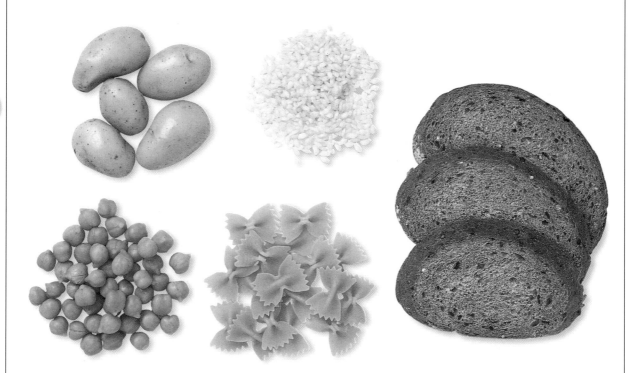

■ **Good sources of complex carbohydrates** *are potatoes, rice, bread, pasta, and garbanzo beans. Not only do these starchy foods supply fiber, but they also satisfy the appetite so you'll feel full longer.*

2 Complex carbohydrates: Also known as starches. Grains and grain products, fruits, vegetables, beans, and dairy products are all sources of complex carbohydrates. Because they are made from more complex molecules, it takes longer for the body to break down these foods. Compared to the sugar "blast," these carbs last.

3 Cellulose: Also known as fiber. This carbohydrate is so exceedingly complex that the human body cannot digest it at all. (Cows and horses can, which is why they are able to fill all of their nutritional needs by eating grass and hay.)

A balanced diet for an adult should draw 55 to 60 percent of its calories from carbohydrates, with the greatest proportion being complex carbohydrates.

INTERNET

www.iVillage.com/ food/tools

To find out what percentage of calories should come from each food group, check out the Health Calculator on the iVillage site. It will ask you a few personal questions and tell you your carbohydrate, fat, and protein RDA and total daily calorie needs.

A WORD ABOUT WATER

Water is essential for digestion, as well as the conversion of food to energy, the elimination of waste, and about a zillion other body functions. You could more easily do without food than water. We'll be talking more later on about the role water plays in diet and health, but for now here's a tip about water and fiber: Soluble fiber dissolves in water; insoluble fiber swells up, increasing the feeling of fullness. That's good. But fiber may cause constipation, and that could be bad. The best way to avoid getting constipated is to drink at least eight 8-ounce glasses of water a day. Since water has zero calories, drink up!

Regardless of whether the carbohydrate is simple or complex, each gram supplies 4 calories. Horses get 4 calories out of their gram of grass, but since we cannot digest fiber, it provides us with zero calories.

Does that mean there's no point in eating fiber? Quite the contrary. Fiber has many benefits. What it lacks in calories it more than makes up in bulk. It gives you a feeling of fullness that helps curb hunger.

Because it is indigestible, fiber sticks around for a long time, so you feel full far longer than you do when you have a sweet snack or sugary drink.

Best of all, fiber lowers blood cholesterol levels and reduces the risk of developing diabetes. It also protects against such intestinal problems as constipation and *diverticulitis*.

You should include 25 to 30 grams of fiber in your daily diet.

Whole grains, beans, nuts, and dried fruit (raisins, prunes, dates, and figs, for example) are all high in fiber.

> **DEFINITION**
>
> *Diverticulitis is a painful condition that occurs when small pouches (diverticula) that form in the wall of the colon are clogged with feces and become inflamed.*

Life's building blocks

PROTEINS ARE COMPLEX COMPOUNDS

made up of amino acids. Often called the "building blocks" of the body, amino acids are used to create, maintain, and repair all protein components of the body. These include body tissues such as skin, hair, bones, muscles, and organs, as well as digestive enzymes, hormones, various components of the immune system, and even genes.

Proteins also supply heat and energy, but not as readily as carbohydrates.

The average adult needs about half a gram of protein per pound of body weight.

Infants need three times as much protein as adults to support their rapid growth, and children need twice the amount.

PROTEIN RDAs*

Infants	up to 12 months	13–14 grams
Children	1–3 years old	16 grams
	4–6 years old	24 grams
	9–10 years old	28 grams
Males	11–14 years old	45 grams
	15–18	59 grams
	19–24	58 grams
	25 and older	63 grams
Females	11–14 years old	46 grams
	15–18	44 grams
	19–24	46 grams
	25 and older	50 grams

*based on average weights

The richest sources of protein are animal foods, especially meat, cheese, and eggs. Protein is also found in some foods of plant origin, especially beans and nuts.

Regardless of a protein's source, how it is grown, processed, or prepared, the calorie count is the same. Every gram of protein contains 4 calories, the same gram for gram, as carbohydrates.

This does not mean that a gram of hamburger meat contains 4 calories. Hamburger and other meats contain both protein and fat. The 4 calories per gram is for pure protein. In fact, all calories per gram figures refer to these nutrients in their pure form. But most of the foods we eat contain combinations of nutrients.

■ **Animal proteins** *are found in meat, fish, and dairy products. Plant proteins, like beans and lentils, are generally healthier because they're lower in fat.*

The skinny on fats

FATS, OR LIPIDS, *are non-water-soluble molecules that the body uses in many different ways. Fats supply immediate energy or can be stored for future use. They are an important component of many body cells. They transport nutrients, including fat-soluble vitamins, and play a key role in normal growth and development. Fats occur naturally in many plants and animals. Oils are pure fats in liquid form that are extracted from plant and animal sources.*

Because of their high calorie content and the health risks associated with them, fats should make up no more than 30 percent of your *daily caloric intake.* (15%)

Many health experts recommend an even smaller percentage, going as low as 10 percent. The body cannot do without any fat at all, but in our culture there is little danger of anyone eating a fat-deficient diet!

Saturated and unsaturated fats

You have undoubtedly heard the terms saturated and unsaturated fats. To keep it simple: *Saturated fats* are solid at room temperature, whereas *unsaturated fats* are liquid. Butter and the fat you see around a piece of steak, for example, are saturated fats. Olive and other vegetable oils are unsaturated fats.

Although saturated fats generally come from animals and unsaturated fats come from plants, there are two exceptions. Coconut and palm (or palm kernel) oils are saturated fats, despite being of plant origin. This is a fact worth paying attention to since many commercial baked goods – cookies, crackers, and the like – are made with coconut or palm oil or both. Read the label before you buy or bite!

No matter whether they are saturated or unsaturated, animal or vegetable, natural, organic, virgin or processed, cold pressed or rendered, all fats provide the same amount of calories: 9 per gram.

How saturated and unsaturated fats differ is in the effect they have on cholesterol levels in your blood.

Saturated fats raise the level of LDL in your blood. And you know what happens to excess LDL. It is deposited on the inner walls of the arteries, leading to atherosclerosis, high blood pressure, and other health problems.

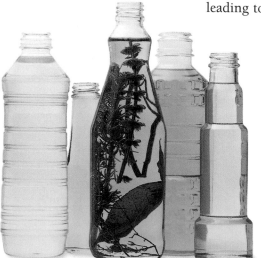

Unsaturated fats, on the other hand, do not increase the level of LDL in your blood. In fact, they lower it! That makes them a valuable addition to your diet. But beware: Even though unsaturated fats perform this cholesterol-lowering service, they still are packed with calories. Like any fat, unsaturated fats contain 9 calories per gram.

■ **Unsaturated fats** *are liquid at room temperature. They won't raise cholesterol but they have as many calories as any other fat.*

CONFUSED ABOUT CHOLESTEROL?

The cholesterol circulating in your blood is called blood, serum, or endogenous, cholesterol. The cholesterol you eat is called dietary cholesterol. There is a difference between the two. Dietary cholesterol comes from animal products: meat, eggs, milk, and other dairy products. Vegetables, nuts, and oils made from them do not contain cholesterol. Although eating foods high in dietary cholesterol will increase the level of your blood cholesterol, food is not the only source of cholesterol, and it is not even the main one.

The liver is your body's cholesterol factory: About 80 percent of the cholesterol circulating in your blood is made by your liver; only 20 percent comes from food. All animals, including humans, make cholesterol in their livers. When you eat animal meat and products of animal origin, you're getting the cholesterol made by their livers. Your liver uses saturated fat in the food you eat to manufacture cholesterol. That's why foods that are high in saturated fat increase the amount of cholesterol your liver sends out to the rest of your body through your blood.

FAT RDA

According to the US Department of Agriculture (USDA), a healthful diet will contain no more than these proportions of fat. That means fat added to or hidden in all the food you eat in a single day.

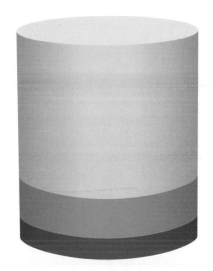

☐ **Total calories**

☐ **Fat:** less than 30 percent of total calories

■ <u>**Saturated fat:**</u> less than 10 percent of total calories

Cholesterol: less than 300 milligrams

Trans fats

I've mentioned butter and oils, but what about margarine? It is an unsaturated fat, made from vegetable oil, but it has been hydrogenated. That means hydrogen atoms have been added to each molecule to "saturate" it so it takes a solid form at room temperature. The added hydrogen atoms also make it more stable, so it is less likely to become rancid.

Sounds good? Well, actually, no. This synthetic saturated fat is called trans fat and the news about it is bad. Long marketed as the low-cholesterol alternative to butter, margarine has recently had a lot of bad press. Most of it is based on a medical study that showed that people whose diets are high in trans fats are at increased risk for heart attack. The risk is related to the fact that trans fats not only raise LDL levels, but also lower levels of HDL, the "good" cholesterol.

One small piece of good news: Liquid margarine, the kind that comes in squeeze bottles, and some tub margarines contain less trans fat than the solid stick kind.

Want to avoid trans fats? As of now, you won't find them listed by that name on food packaging, which is why some people call them "stealth fats," but the USDA is considering new regulations that would require trans fats to be listed. Until such changes are made, you need to look for the words "hydrogenated" and "partially hydrogenated" on the label of all prepared foods you buy.

INTERNET

mayohealth.org

No, this is not the all-the-mayo-you-can-eat web site. The Mayo Clinic Health Oasis is chock-full of valuable health information. Click on "Nutrition" and you will find articles, Q&As, self-assessment tools, tips, and solid facts about eating and weight loss.

■ **French fries,** *potato, and other chips, crackers, and donuts are all major sources of trans fats, as are fast foods. Try to avoid these foods as much as you can.*

What about alcohol?

Is it fat, protein, or carbohydrate? Actually, it's none of the above. It is yet another source of energy – after all, it can be burned to provide light and even to run an automobile – but it's not, strictly speaking, a nutrient. Alcohol supplies 7 calories per gram, about halfway between fats and protein/carbohydrates. It is processed by the liver and turned into fat for storage. That's where beer bellies come from, in case you were wondering.

The mighty micronutrients

VITAMINS AND MINERALS are called micronutrients because we consume and need only tiny amounts of them. A little goes a long way, but having too little also has a great impact.

In a balanced diet such as is available in developed countries, you will probably get all the vitamins and minerals you need. But be aware that I said "balanced diet."

A diet full of junk food or one that ignores one or more of the food groups is not balanced and may well be deficient in some important vitamins and minerals.

If you're living on junk food, don't think that the answer is to pop a vitamin pill and hope for the best. Instead, balance your diet!

Vitamins

Vitamins are major players in the process by which food is broken down and converted to energy or stored as fat. The body also uses vitamins to help manufacture blood cells, hormones, genes, and parts of the nervous system.

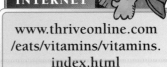

INTERNET

www.thriveonline.com
/eats/vitamins/vitamins.
index.html

This guide is brought to you by Oxygen Media's health channel. Click on a vitamin or mineral to find out what it does, how much you need daily, where to get it in the food you eat, and what goes wrong if you have too little (or too much).

DEFINITION

Oxidation is a process of decay that includes rusting (in metals) and spoilage (in some foods). It is also believed to be involved in some disease processes in humans and other animals. **Antioxidants** *inhibit or prevent oxidation. One such antioxidant is beta carotene, a yellow to red pigment found in many foods and converted to vitamin A by the liver.*

Vitamins are either water-soluble or fat-soluble. The water-soluble vitamins are C and the B group. The fat-soluble vitamins are A, D, E, and K. Beta-carotene, that famous *antioxidant,* is also fat-soluble. Fat-soluble vitamins are found in foods that contain fat, which is one reason why a completely fat-free diet isn't healthy.

Minerals

Minerals are required for many body processes, including making and maintaining bones and soft tissues, keeping the nervous system in operation, and clotting blood. Unlike vitamins, some of which are made by the body, minerals must be supplied by foods or as supplements. Essential minerals are calcium, phosphorus, magnesium, iron, iodine, potassium, copper, cobalt, manganese, fluorine, and zinc. You need traces of other minerals as well.

THE FOOD PYRAMID

The food pyramid is a simple graphic tool developed by the USDA for designing a healthful diet. It shows the relative proportion of the food groups you should eat every day. The operative word is *serving*. In Chapter 9 we will be talking about what a serving is and how to be sure you don't pile your plate with more than one. For now, though, just remember that the food pyramid is about eating a balanced diet. It does not necessarily prescribe a low-calorie one.

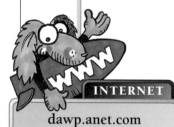

INTERNET

dawp.anet.com

The Diet Analysis Web Page will figure out the amount of calories, protein, and various vitamins and minerals in whatever you eat. Click on the food and the number of servings, enter your gender and age, and back comes a chart or bar graph with the amount of each nutrient and its percentage of the RDA. It includes lots of fast foods by brand.

1 Eat sparingly

Sweets, fats, and oils should make up only a tiny part of your daily diet.

2 Eat 2–3 servings

All meat (including fish), dairy products (except for butter, which has been banished to the top of the food pyramid), beans, and nuts should be consumed in moderation. Animal flesh and eggs are sources of protein and fat. Dairy products are good sources of calcium and some vitamins. They are a mixture of protein, carbohydrate, and fat. Beans and nuts are foods of plant origin that are good sources of carbohydrate, protein, and fiber. Beans tend to be low in fat, whereas nuts are high in fat.

■ **The idea of the food pyramid** *is that the bottom, or widest part, represents the foods you should eat most of, whereas the pointy narrow top tells you to eat very little of the foods up there.*

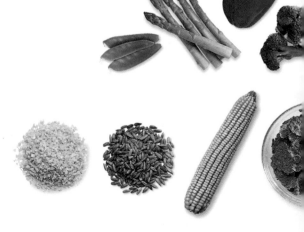

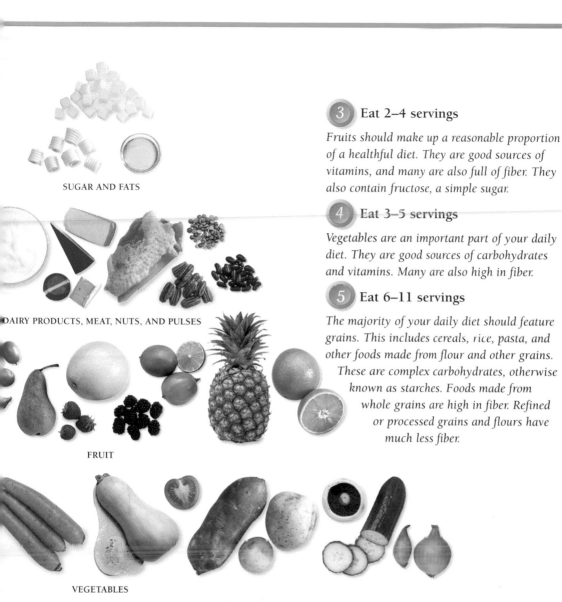

SUGAR AND FATS

DAIRY PRODUCTS, MEAT, NUTS, AND PULSES

FRUIT

VEGETABLES

GRAINS AND CEREALS

3 Eat 2–4 servings

Fruits should make up a reasonable proportion of a healthful diet. They are good sources of vitamins, and many are also full of fiber. They also contain fructose, a simple sugar.

4 Eat 3–5 servings

Vegetables are an important part of your daily diet. They are good sources of carbohydrates and vitamins. Many are also high in fiber.

5 Eat 6–11 servings

The majority of your daily diet should feature grains. This includes cereals, rice, pasta, and other foods made from flour and other grains. These are complex carbohydrates, otherwise known as starches. Foods made from whole grains are high in fiber. Refined or processed grains and flours have much less fiber.

How to read a food label

By law, all packaged and prepared foods must carry nutritional labeling, but how many people actually read the labels? There's a whole lot of valuable information to be found there. Let's look at the label on a box of cookies, for example.

a **Serving size:** If you think an entire box of cookies is a serving, the label will set you straight. A serving, in this case, is three cookies, for a total of 180 calories. If you can eat just one, you've swallowed 60 calories. If you eat all 15, you've scarfed down 900 calories.

b **Fat facts:** If you look hard enough, you'll find a lot of information. "Calories from fat" tells you that, in this case, fully half of each serving is fat. Next, look at the heading "Total Fat." There are 10 grams per serving.

Remember: We're talking about three cookies, not one and certainly not all 15. At 9 calories per gram, that ought to add up to 90 calories . . . yes, that checks out with "calories from fat." But what kind of fat is it? Three types are represented here: saturated, polyunsaturated, and monounsaturated. What about trans fats? These "stealth fats" aren't mentioned by name, but you can do a little math and figure it out:

If total fat is 10 grams, but the sum of the fats listed is 9.5 grams, 0.5 grams are trans fats.

Finally, three cookies contain 10 mg of cholesterol, 3 percent of the maximum you should take in daily.

But, wait, there are more fat facts on the label. Look down at the ingredients and see how many sources of fat you can find there. The obvious ones are the oils: soybean, cottonseed, and/or canola oils. But before you celebrate their being unsaturated vegetable oils, notice the words "partially hydrogenated." This is the source of the trans fats. Can you find other fats in the ingredients? There's the cocoa butter in the chocolate. And the fat in whole eggs. No wonder half the calories come from fat!

c **Other nutrients:** Between the flour and the sugars they are made with, cookies are mainly carbohydrates – 21 grams in all. The label specifies the amount of sugars and fiber, because these are considered most important from the point of view of health, but the two won't add up to the total carbs. The rest are complex carbohydrates.

Nutrition Facts

Serving Size 3 cookies (34g/1.2 oz)

Servings Per Container About 5

Amount Per Serving

Calories 180	Calories from Fat 90

% Daily Value*

Total Fat 10g	**15%**
Saturated Fat 3.5g	**18%**
Polyunsaturated Fat 1g	
Monounsaturated Fat 5g	
Cholesterol 10mg	**3%**
Sodium 80mg	**3%**
Total Carbohydrate 21g	**7%**
Dietary Fiber 1g	**4%**
Sugars 11g	
Protein 2g	

Vitamin A 0%	Vitamin C 0%
Calcium 2%	Iron 4%
Thiamin 6%	Riboflavin 4%
Niacin 4%	

* Percent Daily Values are based on a 2,000 calorie diet. Your daily values may be higher or lower depending on your calorie needs:

	Calories	2,000	2,500
Total Fat	Less than	65g	80g
Sat Fat	Less than	20g	25g
Cholesterol	Less than	300mg	300mg
Sodium	Less than	2,400mg	2,400mg
Total Carbohydrate		300g	375g
Dietary Fiber		25g	30g

Ingredients: Unbleached enriched wheat flour [flour, niacin, reduced iron, thiamin mononitrate (vitamin B$_1$)], sweet chocolate [sugar, chocolate liquor, cocoa butter, soy lecithin added as an emulsifier, vanilla extract], sugar, partially hydrogenated vegetable shortening [soybean, cottonseed and/or canola oils], nonfat milk. whole eggs, cornstarch, egg whites. salt, vanilla extract, baking soda, and soy lecithin.

Serving size *reflects the amount typically eaten by many people*

The list of nutrients *covers those most important to the health of today's consumers*

Calories from Fat *are now shown on the label to help consumers meet dietary guidelines that recommend people get no more than 30 percent of the calories in their overall diet from fat*

% Daily Value (DV) *shows how a food in the specified serving size fits into the overall daily diet. By using the % DV you can easily determine whether a food contributes a lot or a little of a particular nutrient. And you can compare different foods with no need to to do any calculations*

■ **Food labels can** *tell you a great deal, but you have to read them carefully. Look at the serving size, the number of calories from fat, and what types of fats the product contains.*

Even so, 11 grams of sugar is an awful lot. Remember: Sugar is at the top of the pyramid, in the "eat sparingly" department.

Protein is listed, though in the case of cookies, this is a paltry amount. On other food labels, protein might play a bigger part.

 More on ingredients: The earlier in the list an ingredient appears, the more (by weight) there is of it. There are many loopholes to this rule, and manufacturers take advantage of every one. For example, they use a lot of different kinds of sugar. Since each one represents only a very small amount by weight, various sugars can hide toward the end of the ingredients list. To paraphrase the poet, "A sugar by any other name is just as sweet," and still a sugar. Here are some of the aliases sugar goes by:

- brown sugar
- corn sweetener
- corn syrup
- fructose
- fruit juice concentrate
- glucose
- dextrose
- high-fructose corn syrup
- honey
- invert sugar
- lactose
- maltose
- molasses
- raw sugar
- sucrose
- syrup

Because sugar is a carbohydrate, every gram contains 4 calories, no matter what name it travels under. So be as aware of "stealth" sugars as you are of "stealth" fats.

Do yourself a favor and become an avid label reader. You can learn a lot about how much of what is in the food you eat.

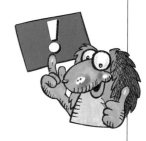

A simple summary

✓ All foods consist of one or more of the three main nutrient types: carbohydrate, protein, and fat.

✓ Both protein and carbohydrate provide 4 calories per gram; each gram of fat provides more than double that: 9 calories. Though not really a nutrient, alcohol provides 7 calories per gram.

✓ A healthful diet gets 55 to 60 percent of its calories from carbohydrates, most of which should be complex carbohydrates (starches) and very few simple carbohydrates (sugars).

✓ Dietary fiber has health benefits and helps curb appetite, so a fiber-rich diet makes sense.

✓ Adults should eat a half-gram of protein for every pound of body weight.

✓ Fats should account for no more than 30 percent of daily caloric intake and preferably less than that.

✓ Saturated fats raise levels of LDL (the "bad" cholesterol), so they should be limited to no more than 10 percent of caloric intake.

✓ Unsaturated fats do not raise LDL levels, and some increase HDL (the "good" cholesterol), so these should be emphasized.

✓ Vitamins and minerals are necessary in small quantities to maintain health and many body functions. The best source of these micronutrients is a balanced diet.

✓ Make it a habit to read food labels carefully, and watch out for hidden fats and sugars in the processed foods you buy.

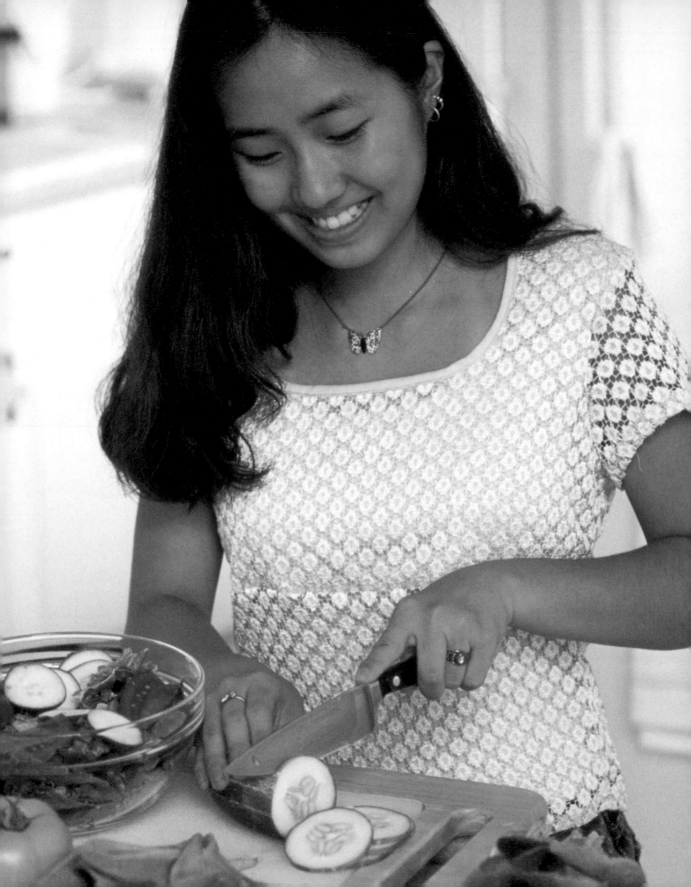

Chapter 5

Why (and How) Calories Count

CALORIES DO COUNT! However pleasurable eating is, its real purpose is to provide the energy your body needs to maintain a constant temperature and perform its basic functions. Anything extra you do uses more calories. Any calories you consume that your body does not need are converted to body fat. It's as simple as that. The goal of this chapter is to help you understand what happens to food after it goes in your mouth. This should combat foolish or dangerous myths about food and weight loss.

In this chapter...

✓ *The meaning of metabolism*

✓ *Calories in*

✓ *Calories out*

✓ *Daily calorie needs*

✓ *Balancing intake and output*

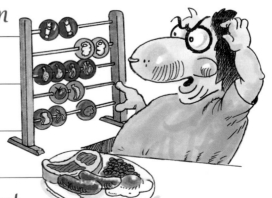

YOU ARE WHAT YOU EAT: CONSUME MORE CALORIES THAN YOU NEED AND YOUR BODY WILL STORE THEM

The meaning of metabolism

METABOLISM IS THE SUM TOTAL OF *all the chemical and physical processes by which the body breaks down, converts, and uses food, gases, and other substances. For our purposes, we will focus on how the body metabolizes food, converting it into forms that can be used immediately – for energy or to build and repair tissues – or stored for future use.*

The digestive system breaks down food into its component parts. Carbohydrates become the simple sugar glucose. Fats are broken down into fatty acids, which are the main type of molecules that make up fats and are not soluble in water. Proteins are broken down into amino acids. These components go to the liver, where they are prepared for use or storage.

Glucose is used immediately for energy or is stored as *glycogen*. But there is a limit to how much glycogen your cells can store. Once the glycogen "bank" is full, the rest is stored as fat. Amino acids are used to build and repair cells, among many other tasks. Anything left over is stored as fat. Fatty acids go straight to the fat cells. Are you beginning to get the picture? Fat cells are the ultimate destination for all nutrients your body does not need for immediate use.

Do not believe any "expert" who claims to have discovered how to change the way your body uses food, or a magic combination of foods that "work together" to burn more calories.

The metabolism meter

The thyroid secretes hormones that regulate metabolism. People with overactive thyroids (hyperthyroidism) will suddenly lose weight, even though their appetites increase. They will also feel nervous and jumpy. This is because their metabolism has been speeded up. Conversely, an underactive thyroid (hypothyroidism) will cause weight gain and a sluggish, low-energy feeling. These are both serious medical conditions that require accurate diagnosis.

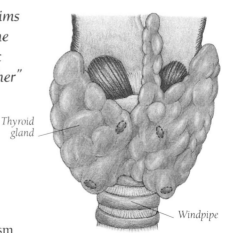

Thyroid gland

Windpipe

■ **The thyroid is a gland** *that wraps around the windpipe in your throat. It secretes hormones that regulate your metabolic rate.*

MORE WATER

The chemical processes involved in metabolism require water. This is yet another reason to be sure you drink enough. Although there is water in much of the food and drink you swallow, it's still important to drink a minimum of two quarts of plain old H_2O every day. Don't wait until you are thirsty to pour yourself a glass. It's thought that the "thirst" message comes when you are already somewhat dehydrated.

Calories in

EVERYBODY TALKS ABOUT CALORIES, but how many people know what a calorie actually is? We tend to think of calories as something "contained in" food, like sugar or fat. In fact, a calorie is a scientific unit of heat measurement.

DEFINITION

A **calorie** is the amount of energy needed to raise the temperature of 1 gram of water by 1° C. Scientists usually work with a larger unit called a kilocalorie (Kcal), which is the amount of energy needed to raise the temperature of a kilogram of water by 1° C. But since it takes exactly 1,000 times more energy to raise the temperature of 1,000 times more water (kilo = 1,000), the number of calories and kilocalories are comparable. To keep it plain and simple, most people use calories when talking about food.

What does all this have to do with food? When food is digested, it is broken down into a form the body can either use or store. When used, it is "burned," giving off heat energy that is measurable in calories. When stored, it is potential energy, energy that is able to be burned at some future time. That too is measurable in calories.

How many calories make a pound of fat? The answer is 3,500, whether they're coming or going.

If you eat 3,500 more calories than your body needs, they will be stored and add a pound to your weight. On the other hand, if you burn 3,500 more calories than you eat, they will be drawn from your fat stores and you'll lose a pound. The good and bad news about this is that your body is a remarkably shrewd accountant. Whether you eat those extra 3,500 in a day, a week, a month, or a year, the deposit will always be a pound. The same goes for the withdrawal.

Just as a reminder, the three major nutrients – carbohydrate, protein, and fat – and the quasinutrient alcohol provide energy to the body that is measurable in calories. This energy can be either used immediately or stored for future use. Their calorie content is as follows:

- **Carbohydrate**: 4 calories per gram
- **Protein**: 4 calories per gram
- **Fat**: 9 calories per gram
- **Alcohol**: 7 calories per gram

Storing the excess

If we expended every bit of energy we take in as food, we'd be a skinny bunch, and this book would be collecting dust along with all the other diet books. We'd also be in big trouble if food became scarce or the weather turned very cold or we got sick, because then we wouldn't have stored fat to draw on. But this is theoretical. Except in parts of the world where famine is reality, most of us help ourselves to more calories than we actually need, and we carry the extra on our hips and elsewhere.

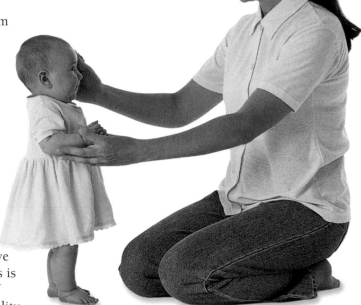

■ **Body fat makes up** *20 to 25 percent of a woman's weight, compared to 15 to 20 percent for a man. Fat deposits are essential for female fertility as they maintain healthy hormone production.*

It doesn't matter whether you eat too much fat, too much carbohydrate, too much protein, or a combination of the three. The body breaks down all the food so it is ready for use or for storage.

Everybody needs some body fat. You need it in the marrow of your bones, where red blood cells are made. You need it around your organs, to cushion them and to keep them warm. Your brain also needs it, your nerves need it, and women particularly need it to keep their reproductive systems working properly. In fact, as much as 50 percent of the fat in your body is used for these essential purposes. The rest is stored directly under your skin, and that's the fat that shows.

There's an important wrinkle in the metabolic process that provides a hint why fat makes you fatter than protein and carbohydrates. It takes considerable energy to fuel the metabolism itself, but it is far easier for the body to metabolize fat than protein or carbohydrate.

Because dietary fat is close to the form it needs to be in for storage, metabolizing it requires just 3 calories for every 100 you eat. That leaves 97 calories to be stored in your fat cells.

Converting carbohydrates to storable fat is a complex process, taking 23 of every 100 calories. Once the conversion has taken place, only 77 calories remain to be stored. Depending on the exact amino acids involved, metabolizing protein requires fewer calories than carbohydrate but more than fat.

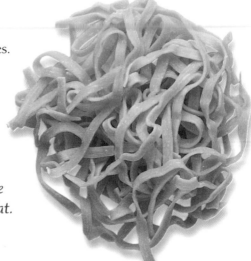

Carbohydrates are your best bet if you want to reduce the amount of excess stored as fat.

People who promote high-fat, high-protein, and low-carbohydrate weight-loss diets are ignoring the basic scientific facts. Now that you know the truth, make sure that you don't fall for their dietary mumbo jumbo.

■ **Eating carbohydrates** *such as pasta and bread is a good idea because your body has to work that much harder to digest them – burning more calories in the process.*

Fat cells are immortal

When you lose weight, the amount of fat stored in the cells is reduced, but the cells themselves stay there, waiting for more storable fat to come along. They do collapse a little, but there's no escaping the fact that they're still there.

Alas, losing weight won't get rid of fat cells, but gaining weight will actually cause your body to make more. That's because each cell can hold only so much fat. If all the existing fat cells are filled to capacity, your body will simply manufacture new ones to cope with the excess.

Trivia...
Did you know that a person whose weight is normal has around 30 billion fat cells? People who are overweight might have as many as 100 billion fat cells, and a severely obese person could host as many as 270 billion!

Calories out

WHEN YOU THINK ABOUT EXPENDING ENERGY, you probably think about your daily activities, but a full 60 percent of the energy that your body uses is devoted to basic life functions. It takes energy – lots of it – to keep your heart beating, your lungs working, your brain ticking, and especially to keep your temperature at 98.6° F.

The process of expending energy for basic body processes alone – with no extra physical activities factored in – is called your basal metabolism. The rate at which this energy is expended is your basal metabolic rate (BMR). As a rule, basal metabolism consumes 10 calories for every pound of a woman's body weight and 11 calories per pound for men. A woman who weighs 140 pounds, for example, expends 1,400 calories just to run her body. That's without lifting a finger or walking an inch. A 140-pound man would burn 1,540 calories. It may not be fair, but that's the way it is.

If that woman sat in a chair all day and ate no more nor less than 1,400 calories, she would neither gain nor lose weight. On 1,800 calories, she'd gain weight; on 1,200 calories, she'd lose. Either way, she'd be bored.

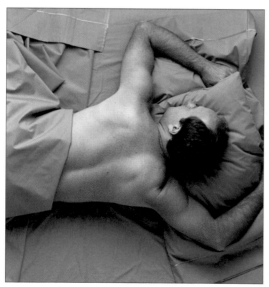

■ **Even when we're asleep** *our bodies are using energy, although it's only a tiny amount.*

The heavier a person is, the greater the need for calories. A 200-pound woman, who might be very overweight, would require 2,000 calories for basal metabolism alone. (A man of the same weight would need 2,200 calories.) This means that weight loss should be easier for a heavier person: just cut back to 1,500 calories and lose a pound a week. Add a little activity, say a half-hour walk at a snail's pace of 2 mph, and the same woman can eat 1,600 calories a day and still lose that pound a week.

Now, a person who is overweight probably eats far in excess of daily needs. Cutting back to 1,500 to 1,600 calories may be easier to say than do, and that half-hour walk would be a challenge. But these are goals worth aiming for.

Speeding up or slowing down your BMR

The greater the proportion of your total body weight that is represented by muscles, the higher your BMR. Muscle cells are eight times more metabolically active than fat cells.

Plain and simple, more muscular people require more calories to run their bodies. How's that for a motivator!

There's another wrinkle in the BMR picture. As we age, our energy needs decrease. On average, it drops 2 percent per decade. Remember, we lose muscle mass as we age. That's one reason why older people need fewer calories. It's also why, if they continue to eat the same amount they always have, people tend to get heavier as they grow older. This is compounded if they also cut back on activity, either because of ill health or a misguided notion that their active days are behind them.

Several fad diets and many "diet aids" claim to be able to speed up metabolism so you burn calories more efficiently. Some of them don't work, and those that do can be hazardous to your health. But there is a perfectly natural, perfectly healthy way to speed up your metabolism. It's by being more active.

■ **A muscular person** *weighing about 200 pounds would have a much higher calorie requirement for basal metabolism than an unfit person of the same weight. This is because, ounce for ounce and pound for pound, muscles burn more energy than fat.*

Trivia...

Why can some people eat what they like and not gain weight? It turns out these folks have naturally speedy metabolisms. Scientists investigating nonexercise activity thermogenesis (NEAT) have found that the metabolic rate in people with high rates of NEAT increased markedly after a high-calorie meal. Why some people are NEATer than others isn't clear. It may be connected to hormones or genetics.

Exercise boosts your BMR and keeps it up for as long as 12 hours after you stop sweating.

An hour-long workout at the gym will rev up your BMR for the rest of the day or longer, and all the while you'll be burning calories at a faster rate. Can anything slow your BMR? Yes. Aside from age and inactivity, dieting will do just that. That may sound backward, but the fact is, your body has fairly primitive responses. When you eat less, it interprets the reduced caloric intake as a sign of famine. So, it slows down the BMR to decrease energy needs. This is the scientific explanation behind weight-loss plateaus and the set point (to be discussed in Chapter 6.)

Daily calorie needs

IF YOU WANT TO MAINTAIN YOUR WEIGHT, you must take in neither more nor fewer calories than your body needs to maintain basic metabolism and to fuel any additional activity. If you want to lose weight, you must take in fewer calories than needed. You can do this by eating less, being more active, or better, a combination of both.

You will lose 1 pound for every 3,500 calories you are in debt to your body. If your daily intake is 35 calories less than your output, it will take you 100 days to lose that pound. Reduce your intake or increase your output by 350 calories daily and it will take 10 days to lose that pound.

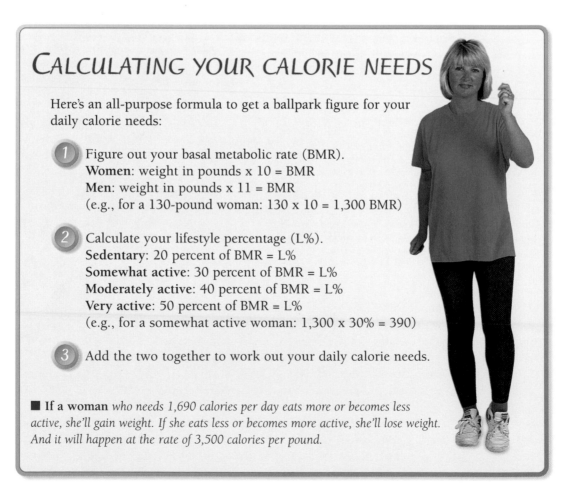

CALCULATING YOUR CALORIE NEEDS

Here's an all-purpose formula to get a ballpark figure for your daily calorie needs:

1. Figure out your basal metabolic rate (BMR).
   Women: weight in pounds x 10 = BMR
   Men: weight in pounds x 11 = BMR
   (e.g., for a 130-pound woman: 130 x 10 = 1,300 BMR)

2. Calculate your lifestyle percentage (L%).
   Sedentary: 20 percent of BMR = L%
   Somewhat active: 30 percent of BMR = L%
   Moderately active: 40 percent of BMR = L%
   Very active: 50 percent of BMR = L%
   (e.g., for a somewhat active woman: 1,300 x 30% = 390)

3. Add the two together to work out your daily calorie needs.

■ *If a woman who needs 1,690 calories per day eats more or becomes less active, she'll gain weight. If she eats less or becomes more active, she'll lose weight. And it will happen at the rate of 3,500 calories per pound.*

The digestion bonus

One of the metabolic processes your body spends energy on is digesting the food you eat. That's right, it takes energy to make energy. As you know, different nutrients take different amounts of energy to digest, but on average 10 percent of your daily energy is spent on digestion.

Just because you expend energy on digestion doesn't mean you should eat more as a way to burn more calories. (Nice try.)

You shouldn't eat more overall, but there is a definitely a case for eating more frequent but smaller meals. Digesting four to six small meals a day burns more calories than digesting three big ones.

Just bear in mind that calories still count. If the four to six small meals contain more calories than the three larger ones, all those extra calories have to be burned with activity or they will be stored you-know-where.

Balancing intake and output

IDEALLY, ANY FITNESS and weight-loss program balances caloric intake and output. No matter how much or how little weight you want to lose, cutting calories alone just won't do it. Not long after it "figures out" that you are taking in fewer calories, your body will respond by decreasing calorie demand. In its wisdom, your body is trying to balance intake and output. The only way to "fool" your body is to increase your level of activity.

The nifty thing about that is you get two for your money when you exercise more. Not only does the energy expenditure burn calories, but your metabolic rate increases, burning even more. If you have been leading a sedentary lifestyle, this does not mean you have to become an exercise freak. Begin with a little more exercise, but do it every day. Gradually add on time or intensity or both.

Stepping up activity even one notch will tell your body to speed up metabolism by about 10 percent.

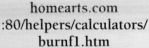

INTERNET

homearts.com
:80/helpers/calculators/
burnf1.htm

Click on this Burn Barometer to find out which activities burn the most calories. Pick the ones you like best and see what they'll do for you. The list runs from aerobics to yoga, with everything from housework and bowling to canoeing and sex in between.

HOW DIFFERENT SPORTS BURN CALORIES

If you're wondering how to add physical activity to your calorie needs ledger, here are some ideas, along with the average number of calories they burn. Be aware, though, that these are approximate figures (assuming an average weight of 150 pounds), since the number of calories burned depends on the intensity of the exercise and your own personal statistics: height, weight, BMI, age, gender, and BMR.

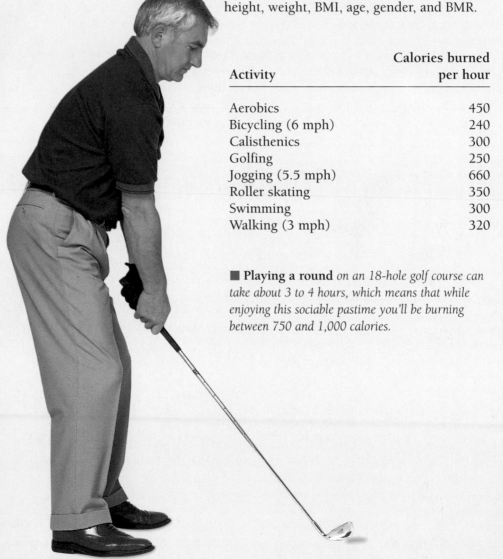

Activity	Calories burned per hour
Aerobics	450
Bicycling (6 mph)	240
Calisthenics	300
Golfing	250
Jogging (5.5 mph)	660
Roller skating	350
Swimming	300
Walking (3 mph)	320

■ **Playing a round** *on an 18-hole golf course can take about 3 to 4 hours, which means that while enjoying this sociable pastime you'll be burning between 750 and 1,000 calories.*

However active you are, there is normally room for improvement, so remember:

1 If you've been sedentary, try to become somewhat active.

2 If you've been somewhat active, try to become moderately active.

3 If you've been moderately active, try to become very active.

4 If you've been very active, keep it up.

When you start being more active, don't overdo it.

If you have been a major couch potato, don't throw yourself into activity with abandon. You may wake up the next day with a serious charley horse or worse, and you will certainly not be able to sustain that level of activity. Start modestly and work your way up to a reasonable level over the course of several weeks or a month. Let it become a habit you don't want to break.

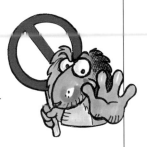

A simple summary

✓ When it comes to gaining or losing weight, calories are what really counts.

✓ Your basal metabolic rate (BMR) is the rate at which your body expends energy (calories) to maintain basic life processes.

✓ Your daily calorie needs depend on your weight, age, gender, and level of activity.

✓ Every pound of body weight represents about 3,500 calories. You must burn 3,500 as energy in order to lose a pound. If you take in 3,500 more calories than you use, you will gain a pound.

✓ Calories in excess of your body's energy needs are stored, mostly as fat, for future use.

✓ Muscle burns eight times more energy than fat. The more muscular you are, the higher your BMR.

✓ Restricting calories slows your metabolism, making it difficult to sustain weight loss by diet alone.

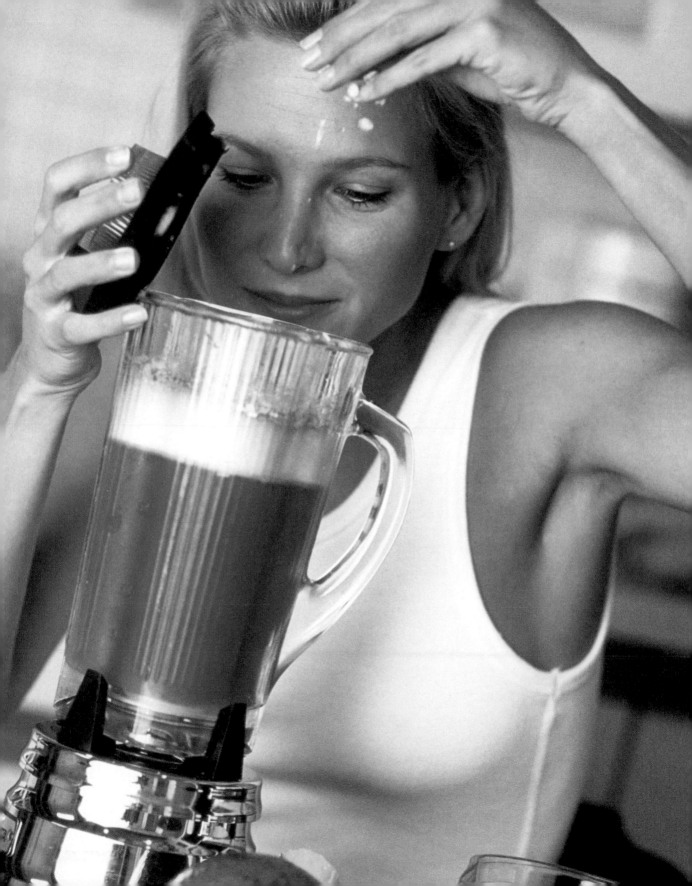

Chapter 6

Weight Loss Questions Answered

THERE ARE PROBABLY MORE MYTHS and misconceptions about weight loss than there are solid facts. Let's take a look at some of the questionable claims about weight loss made in other diet books and on weight-loss products, and try to separate fact from fiction.

In this chapter...

✓ Can you boost metabolism?

✓ Why does weight loss slow up?

✓ Do drugs and fat burners work?

✓ Is it true that fat fights fat?

✓ Can you spot-reduce?

✓ Can you shrink the stomach?

✓ Am I losing weight or water?

✓ What about genetics?

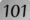

A BALANCED DIET IS ESSENTIAL FOR HEALTH: BEWARE OF DIETS THAT SUGGEST OTHERWISE

Can you boost metabolism?

IN CHAPTER 5, *you learned about metabolism and the role it plays in eating and weight loss. You know that the thyroid gland is your body's metabolism meter. Although there are metabolism boosters on the market, the only safe way to speed up your metabolism is through exercise.*

Unsafe metabolism boosters

There are several diet supplements sold in health food and vitamin stores, through the mail, and on the Internet that claim to speed up metabolism. Some of these are just plain useless, others are downright dangerous.

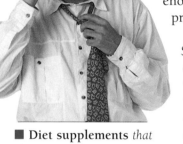

The trouble with these preparations is that they are not regulated by the Food and Drug Administration (FDA), the federal agency that verifies the safety and effectiveness of prescription drugs. As long as they do not make claims to cure a disease, the manufacturers of these products can advertise and sell them to gullible consumers. From time to time, enough cases of harm come to the attention of authorities that a product is taken off the market – but others soon take its place.

■ **Diet supplements** *that claim to speed up metabolism can be dangerous. They may also cause side effects such as nervousness and sweating.*

Some over-the-counter weight-loss supplements contain thyroid extract from animals or other substances that act like the thyroid hormone. These speed metabolism by artificially producing hyperthyroidism. People who take these preparations do lose weight, but they also develop other symptoms of an overactive thyroid, including nervousness and tremor, diarrhea, bulging eyes, racing heartbeat, excessive sweating, and heat intolerance. The FDA is trying to get at least one of these products off the market, warning that it can cause heart attack, stroke, and other serious medical problems.

Do not swallow anything – not the claim, not the product – that says it will speed your metabolism. You are wasting your money or jeopardizing your health or both!

A safe alternative

The only way to safely and effectively increase your metabolic rate is with exercise. The harder you work, the faster your metabolic rate. This is nature's way of responding to increased energy demand. A vigorous exercise session will raise your BMR for many hours. There are so many health and weight-loss benefits to this approach that it's hard to understand why anyone would try anything else.

CHROMIUM PICOLINATE AND EPHEDRA

According to its promoters, chromium picolinate both lowers cholesterol and increases "fat-burning" metabolism. Neither of these claims has withstood scientific study comparing the substance with a placebo (dummy pill).

Chromium picolinate is a synthetic form of chromium, an essential trace mineral abundantly available in most foods. Chromium plays a role in fat metabolism, but no one needs extra amounts.

Excess chromium picolinate can cause flushing, nervousness, and palpitations. It can also cause iron deficiency.

Ephedra is an herbal extract also called *Ma huang*. It may be a "natural" substance, but its active ingredients, ephedrine and pseudoephedrine, are chemicals that have a strong effect on the body. They suppress appetite by stimulating both the nervous system and the thyroid gland. They also cause your air passages to widen, which is why ephedra is promoted as a "natural" decongestant. Among the side effects of ephedra are numbness in the hands and feet due to constriction of blood vessels, elevation of blood pressure, nervousness, and palpitations.

But the problems with ephedra and other thyroid stimulators go beyond their side effects. If you have a healthy thyroid, it doesn't need stimulating. If you have an underactive thyroid, you should see a doctor. It's as simple as that.

Also, don't be swayed by claims that a product is "natural" or "herbal." Regardless of its source or how it is made, once a substance has been metabolized by the body, it acts like the chemical it is.

"Natural" herbs and medicinals are no safer than those made by pharmaceutical companies, and in many cases they are less safe.

If you are buying supplements, always read labels carefully and avoid all products that contain chromium picolinate or ephedra.

Why does weight loss slow up?

ONE OF THE MOST DISCOURAGING THINGS *about trying to lose weight is hitting the plateau. Typically, you start out on a diet filled with determination. Your efforts pay off almost immediately as you rapidly drop a few pounds. And then, a few weeks to a month into your diet, the weight loss slows or even grinds to a halt.*

You have probably heard many explanations for this phenomenon: "The initial weight loss was just water." "The last pounds on are the first pounds off." "You now weigh as much as nature intended." And more.

The set point

Some theorists say every individual has a personal metabolic rate that maintains a given weight, regardless of caloric intake. That personal "ideal" weight, called the set point, is thought to be predetermined by the hypothalamus, an area deep in the brain.

Although the set point theory is based on scientific fact, the mechanism involved is still not fully understood. It has also been oversimplified and often distorted by people promoting a particular diet.

If the set point were really as simple as it sounds, gaining weight would be as difficult as losing it. And we all know that isn't true.

INTERNET

wellweb.com /nutri/fdaart.htm

Click here to read the FDA Guide to Dieting, a no-nonsense article containing the facts on set point and a lot more about the science of weight loss and gain.

At the heart of the set point theory and of the plateau phenomenon is your body's response to calorie restriction. It may be the new millennium, but the human body responds to outside stimuli the same way it did when we were hunting the woolly mammoth. In the face of danger, it secretes extra adrenaline to trigger the "fight or flight" instinct. And in the face of food shortages, it slows down metabolism to protect against starvation during the coming "famine."

You've lost those first few pounds because you're eating less than you need and your body has drawn on your emergency fat stores to make up the difference. It "knows" that once all the glycogen and fat are gone, it will have to start on your muscles, and that would be a disaster. (Muscle wasting is seen in victims of starvation.) You may be far from depleting all of your fat, but your body has no way of knowing how long this "famine" will last, so it plans ahead. It makes your body a more efficient energy consumer to preserve the fat you have on deposit. Thanks a lot! If you reduce your calorie intake even further, you may lose a bit more weight, but it will be hard going and gradually your body will adjust to the new calorie ration and slow down even more. This is a real low point in any weight-loss diet, and it's the time when many people give up.

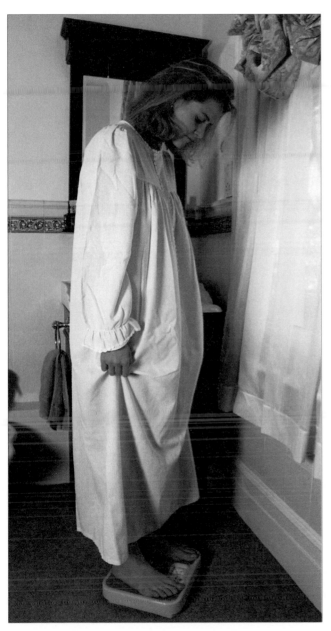

You have no energy, you're hungry, you feel deprived, and you don't seem to be losing any weight. A hot fudge sundae starts looking awfully attractive right about now. Luckily, there's a simple way to "fool" your body and jump off that plateau. You already know what it is, don't you?

Boost your activity level, and you will boost your metabolism.

Add a few minutes to your daily workout, up the intensity, and before you know it, you'll be losing pounds again. As I've already said, you get a double bonus when you do this, since the extra activity will burn calories at the same time it revs up your metabolism.

■ **After losing the first** *few pounds quickly, many people see their weight loss slow down. Exercise more and you'll start to lose weight again as your metabolic rate increases.*

Do drugs and fat burners work?

THERE ARE A LOT OF WEIGHT-LOSS DRUGS

available, both prescription and over-the-counter. There used to be more, but they were banned because of the serious health problems they caused.

Amphetamines and caffeine (far in excess of the dose in your morning cup of coffee) have also been used and discarded as unsafe. Not only do their appetite-suppressing effects eventually wear off over time, but they are harmful to the body. Years ago there was even a diet pill that contained live tapeworm segments that latched onto the gut and helped themselves to the nutrients before the body could absorb them. Yuck!

Prescription drugs

You probably remember phenfen, the combination diet drug that worked by suppressing appetite in the brain (the phen) and speeding metabolism (the fen). Fenfluramine (sold as Pondimin) and dexfenfluramine (sold as Redux) were both withdrawn from the market after it was found that they damaged the heart valves. Phentermine (brand names AdipexP, Fastin, Ionamin, and Obytrim) is still

■ **Appetite suppressors** *cause a host of side effects, including headaches, dizziness, dry mouth, fatigue, insomnia, nausea, and trembling. More seriously, they may increase blood pressure and cause chest pain, urinary retention, fever, hair loss, depression and other mood changes, impotence, and allergic reactions.*

available by prescription, as are five other drugs: orlistat (brand name Xenical), sibutramine (brand name Meridia), diethylproprion (brand names Tenuate and Tepanil), mazindol (brand names Sanorex and Mazanor), and phendimetrazine (brand names Bontril, Plegine, Prelu2, and XTrozine). All of the approved drugs are intended only for people whose BMI is 30 or more (or 27 if they have diabetes, high blood pressure, and/or high cholesterol). And all should be used in partnership with a low-fat diet and exercise.

Orlistat works by blocking fat absorption. This does not mean you can eat all the fat you want and not suffer the consequences.

Orlistat makes most of the fat you eat simply pass along to the intestines for disposal. Some of its unpleasant side effects include frequent, urgent, and oily bowel movements; leakage of oily residue from the rectum; and gas. The more fat you eat, the worse these side effects are.

Blocking fat absorption, as Orlistat does, blocks absorption of essential fat-soluble vitamins, so people who take this drug may be deficient in vitamins A, D, E, and K, and beta carotene.

The other drugs all work by suppressing appetite. All but sibutramine work only for a short time. Within 3 to 12 weeks the brain develops a tolerance for their appetite-suppressing action. Only sibutramine is meant for long-term use.

Do not take any diet drug unless your doctor prescribes it for you, and certainly don't take diet drugs without your doctor's knowledge.

All diet drugs have side effects, some of which are potentially harmful to your health. Their use must be monitored carefully by a doctor or other medical professional. Needless to say, none of these drugs should be taken during pregnancy.

Over-the-counter formulas

Nonprescription diet pills sold as "dietary supplements" are not subject to FDA approval as long as they do not claim to treat a disease. Their safety and effectiveness have not been tested. The chance is great that some terrible side effect will surface in the future. Over the years enough "miracle pills" have turned out to be nightmares that it hardly seems worth the risk.

The latest example is a Chinese herb called *Aristolochia fangchi*, which was given to patients at a Belgian weight-loss clinic. Within three years, more than 100 patients had kidney damage. Many of them needed dialysis or kidney transplants. Now, nearly 10 years after taking the herb, these patients are developing urinary tract cancers. The lesson to be learned from this horrifying story is that it often takes a long time for these kinds of problems to surface when a medicinal product is not subject to clinical trial before it is approved for use. And that is exactly the case with nonprescription dietary supplements.

There are too many such products to list, let alone discuss in detail. My advice is to simply avoid them all.

INTERNET

vm.cfsan.fda.gov/~DMS /aems.html

The FDA's Center for Food Safety and Applied Nutrition, Office of Special Nutritionals, has a web site that will tell you everything you want to know about potentially unpleasant or dangerous side effects of over-the-counter weight-loss and other diet supplements. You can search by ingredient or product name and find out if any problems have been reported for preparations you've heard about and might be considering trying.

Are there fat-burning foods?

No. You may be able to burn fat in a frying pan if you leave it too long on high heat, but the only way to "burn" fat in your body is to expend more energy than is available as glucose in your blood.

Remember when we talked about how excess calories are stored, back in Chapter 5? Carbohydrates are converted to glucose, and that is what is used to provide energy. Excess is stored in your liver and muscles as glycogen, which can be converted back to glucose when needed. When the glycogen storage cells are full, the rest is stored as fatty acid in fat cells. Fat is also stored as fatty acid in fat cells and so is any excess from the protein you eat that is not needed for cell building.

Your body uses the easiest and most available source of energy first. That's glucose. Next it draws on the glycogen and fat storehouses. It uses these two at the same time and in about equal proportions as a way of ensuring that glycogen is not fully depleted.

Any physical activity that requires energy in excess of available glucose will burn fat. The longer and the more intensely you exercise, the more fat you will burn. The scientific principle at work here is nothing more nor less than "calories in, calories out." There are no specific foods, or exercises for that matter, that burn fat more effectively or efficiently than others.

"Fat catalysts"

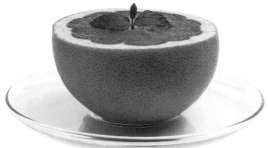

One diet claims to "burn" extra calories because of some magic "catalytic" property found in grapefruit. Now, grapefruit is a wonderful food. It has lots of vitamin C, a decent amount of fiber, and half of a medium fruit has only 50 calories. It is refreshing and delicious and makes a good low-cal snack, dessert, or appetizer, especially if you don't sprinkle it with sugar. But it has no magic properties.

■ **Fresh grapefruit** *makes a delicious, low-calorie breakfast or snack, but it doesn't work miracles; no food is capable of "burning fat."*

The U.S. Postal Service has targeted mail order sales of "grapefruit diet pills" as a prime example of mail fraud. These pills actually contain one or more questionable ingredients that have nothing to do with grapefruit: a diuretic to remove water from your body; glucomannan, a food thickener that can cause intestinal obstruction; and an appetite suppressant that can cause jitteriness and an irregular heartbeat.

Just say "no" to grapefruit diet pills; they do more harm than good.

Is it true that fat fights fat?

UNLESS YOU'VE SPENT *the last few years on Mars, you know about the high-fat, low-carbohydrate diets that have given bacon a new lease on life. I'll be talking more about what's wrong with these diets and why they won't work in the long run in Chapter 10. For now, let me tell you about their immediate, and quite unpleasant, effects.*

The theory behind these diets is that in the absence of carbohydrates, your body concentrates on burning fat. Eating lots of fat is considered fuel for the fire. What's really happening is that the shortage of carbohydrates interferes with complete metabolism of the fats, resulting in a buildup of substances called **ketones**. One of the ketones is acetone, the main ingredient in nail polish remover! If you know anyone on a high-fat, low-carb diet you may have caught a whiff of some really foul "nail polish" breath.

There is no arguing that these diets produce a large initial weight loss, but it's not from the burning of stored fat. It's mostly water loss as the kidneys work overtime to flush out the ketones.

In addition to having bad breath, people on high-fat, low-carb diets are very thirsty. But worse, their body's chemical balance is thrown out of whack.

Ketosis is not a natural state of being; it is a sign that something is wrong metabolically. It is particularly dangerous for people at risk for or with full-blown diabetes. They can go into shock or even die from it.

A high-fat diet can be dangerous for anyone; for people with diabetes, it could be fatal.

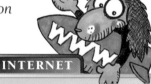

Can you spot-reduce?

YEARS AGO GYMS AND HEALTH CLUBS *were equipped with "exercise" machines that consisted of a motor and a wide canvas strap that you put around your buttocks, stomach, hips, or wherever you felt chubby. The idea was that the vibrating strap was "burning" fat off those specific areas. Guess what? It didn't work.*

Neither do exercises that concentrate on a specific area of the body. That's simply not the way fat cell usage works.

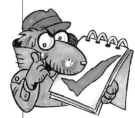

Lifting weights with your arms will strengthen the specific arm muscles you are using, but they will not reduce pockets of fat around or near those muscles.

Where a person loses fat is highly individual. When I lose a few pounds, for example, it first begins to show on my face. Unfortunately, I already have a thin face to offset my ample thighs. But that's the way it is.

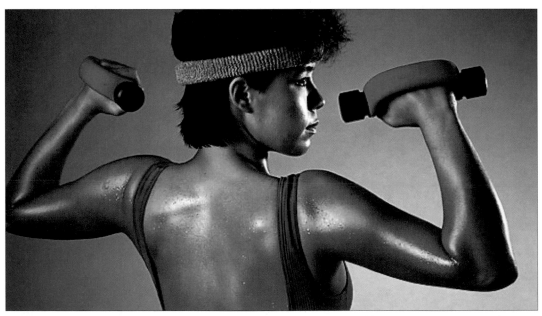

■ **Lifting weights** *improves muscle tone. It will not remove deposits of fat from a targeted part of the body but it will help to firm up flabby areas.*

There is no question that the trimmer, tighter look you get from strength training and other exercise comes from increased muscle tone. A flabby stomach will look flatter when abdominal muscles are strengthened, for example. A tight gluteus maximus will lift even the flabbiest buttocks. But if you are heavy in the hips and you lose 10 pounds, there is no promise that all or even most of the fat will come off your hips.

Liposuction

The only way to remove fat from specific areas of the body is through liposuction, a serious surgical procedure that involves suctioning small pockets of fat from beneath the skin. It is done while you are awake, but a local anesthetic numbs the target area.

Recovery from liposuction can be painful and people who have it may suffer complications, either from the procedure itself or as a reaction to the anesthetic. Bleeding, bruising, and swelling are common, and they may last for weeks or even months. Complications are most common in the very people who need to lose weight and thus might be tempted to try it: those with diabetes, heart disease, and poor circulation.

In some rare instances, people have even died after having liposuction.

Liposuction is also very expensive, and because it is considered cosmetic surgery, few health insurers will pay for it. Still, it is the most popular cosmetic surgery performed in the United States.

But the main problem with liposuction is that if you do not change your eating and exercise habits, your body will quickly replace the fat that was vacuumed away.

Liposuction is not – and never will be – a weight-loss strategy.

Remember: Fat cells are immortal, and if you do not have enough cells to store the excess you eat, your body will obligingly make more. Liposuction is also not a fitness strategy. It will do nothing for your stamina, strength, flexibility, or cardiovascular health.

Trivia...

There's no such thing as cellulite! An entire pseudo-science has grown up around this mythical tissue. The theory is that cellulite is not fat, it's not muscle … it's some sort of "other" that women especially have on their hips and thighs. Search for "cellulite" on the Internet, and you'll find hundreds of sites eager to sell you the newest cellulite buster. What you won't find is a single citation from a medical journal or textbook. That's because, from a medical point of view, cellulite doesn't exist. That pucker is neither more nor less than ripples of fat cells and fibrous connective tissue under the skin. As you get older, your skin's underlying tissue structures become thinner and less elastic. Those are the simple facts; cellulite is a fiction.

Can you shrink the stomach?

YOUR STOMACH IS A MUSCULAR ORGAN *about the size of your hand. Like all muscles, it is resilient: It stretches when it is full and returns to its original size when it is empty.*

You can neither permanently shrink nor stretch your stomach by the amount of food you eat.

As it turns out, both hunger and the feeling of "fullness," or satiety, originate in the brain, not the stomach. Appetite is regulated by the hypothalamus area of the brain, which is how one class of weight-loss drugs works. It is also why mood affects appetite.

The amount of food people eat is largely a matter of habit. It is entirely possible to ignore your brain when it says "Enough!" Compulsive eaters may even have a defect in their "stop eating" brain chemicals.

Still, there are many strategies to control appetite and insure against overeating. We'll be talking about some of them in Chapters 15 and 18. But for now, think about changing habits, rather than shrinking your stomach.

Stomach surgery

These are extreme treatments for life-threatening obesity for which nothing else has worked. People who are morbidly obese who have tried medically supervised diet and exercise, and even prescription diet drugs, but are still unable to lose enough weight may be candidates for gastric surgery.

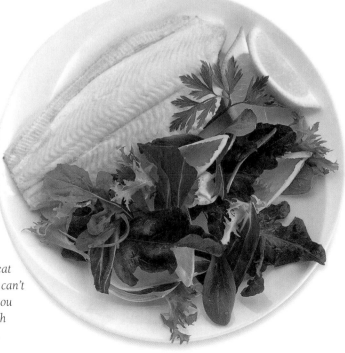

■ **Many people** *who are overweight eat large amounts of food out of habit. You can't shrink the stomach by eating less, but you can lose weight by filling your plate with healthy, rather than high-calorie, foods.*

There are surgical procedures that reduce the size of the stomach. Called gastric restriction or gastric bypass, these either close off all but a small pocket of the stomach or provide a direct passage for food from the esophagus to the intestines, bypassing the stomach.

Surgical procedures are not without risks or expense. Sometimes people develop hernias or gallstones. Anemia and other problems related to nutritional deficiencies are also common. And sometimes the surgical "staples" come out of place. Even when everything works, the procedure requires hospitalization, general anesthesia, and a lengthy period of recovery. Furthermore, people who have had this surgery must still watch their caloric intake and should add exercise to their daily routine. They also require lifelong medical monitoring.

So if you're looking for an easy surgical solution to your munchies problem, this isn't it.

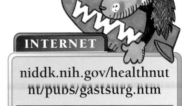

INTERNET

niddk.nih.gov/healthnut
nt/pubs/gastsurg.htm

If you want to know all the gory details of gastric surgery, the National Institute of Diabetes and Digestive and Kidney Diseases has an online pamphlet at this site.

Am I losing weight or water?

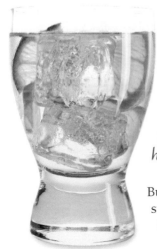

YOU ARE LOSING BOTH. *When stored glycogen is converted to glucose for energy, it releases three parts water for every one part glucose. The glucose is used for energy and the water is excreted in urine.*

Water is pretty heavy stuff. Every fluid ounce weighs about an ounce, so a cup weighs about half a pound. (That makes it simple to remember!)

■ **Drinking lots** *of water is good for you – it helps flush toxins from the body.*

But if you are losing a lot of water weight, you have to be sure to replace it. Drinking more water won't make you fat, but it will replace the water lost during the "breakdown" phase of metabolism. And it will help carry away the waste products. Drinking lots of water is especially important when weight loss is rapid, or when you are increasing activity and losing additional water through sweat. But it is a good idea for everyone.

What about genetics?

"FAT JUST SEEMS TO RUN IN MY FAMILY." *"Everyone on my mother's side is thin, but my father's side of the family is overweight." "I can't do anything about my weight. It's genetic!" You've undoubtedly heard people blame their overweight on genetics, and maybe you've done this yourself.*

Although it is true that genes contribute to BMR, body type, and other factors that influence weight, no one is doomed to obesity by genetics.

Diet, exercise, and other lifestyle habits also "run in families," but they have nothing to do with genes. These are behaviors children pick up and carry into adulthood, and then pass along to their children. If your family has a history of sitting around and eating junk food, that probably explains the "family fat." If, on the other hand, your family history includes sports and other outdoor activities, you and your relatives may all be slim and trim.

You cannot change your genes, but you can change your eating and exercise habits.

Especially if there is a tendency to overweight or weight-related health problems in your family, you should cut down on fats, eat a balanced diet with plenty of complex carbohydrates, and incorporate a minimum of 30 minutes of moderate exercise into every day.

Trivia...

Scientists have found a genetic defect in mice that gives them blond bellies and makes them fat. The defect interferes with a number of hormones and brain chemicals, including some that regulate appetite and fat storage. When injected with a compound that changes the way one brain chemical behaves, the mice quickly lost weight as well as their blondness. The researchers hope to use what they learn from the mice to understand obesity in humans and to develop more effective drug treatments.

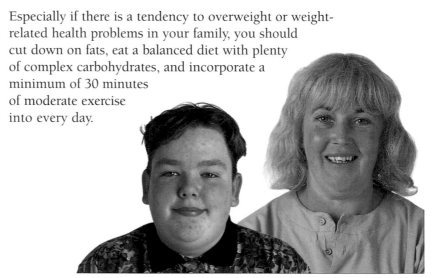

■ **Genes influence** *body type and shape, but lifestyle is a major factor. If being overweight runs in your family, you need to take special care to avoid weight gain yourself.*

If you are overweight, you should begin a program to lose weight and maintain that loss. And if you have children, you should set a good example. Simply put: Healthy living, including eating wisely and being active, can run in families too.

A simple summary

✓ Increased physical activity is the simple answer to most questions about weight loss: It burns calories, boosts metabolism, and gets you off frustrating weight-loss plateaus.

✓ Nonprescription diet pills and other aids are ineffective, dangerous, or both. Because they are not regulated by the FDA, their safety and effectiveness cannot be verified.

✓ Prescription weight-loss drugs are intended only for severely overweight people. They must be part of a medically supervised program that includes a low-fat, low-calorie diet and physical exercise.

✓ Diets that claim to alter the way your body processes food or to rely on special chemical reactions between foods are bogus. Any weight lost on these diets is through calorie restriction.

✓ High-fat, low-carbohydrate diets are unbalanced and unhealthy. They cause chemical changes in your body that can lead to serious health problems.

✓ Neither diet nor exercise will help you "spot reduce." Strengthening and toning muscles may give you a trimmer appearance.

✓ Surgical solutions to overweight are last-ditch solutions that can be risky.

✓ The best way to achieve and maintain a healthy weight is by eating sensibly and being active. This is not a "quick fix." It's a lifetime habit.

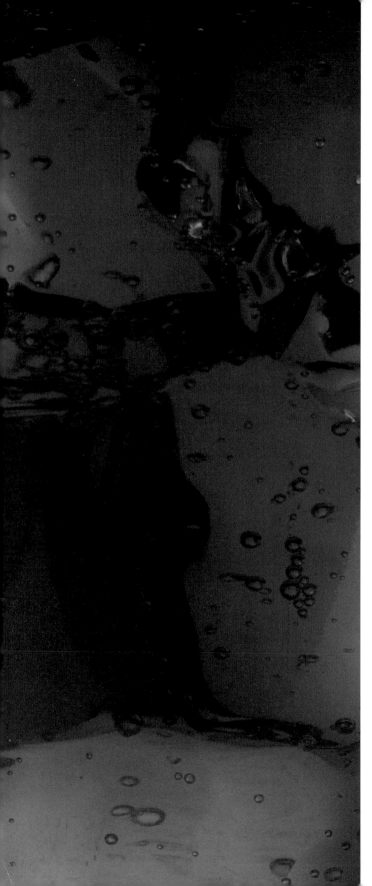

PART THREE

MANY SOFT DRINKS ARE PACKED WITH SUGAR

LOOKING AT YOURSELF

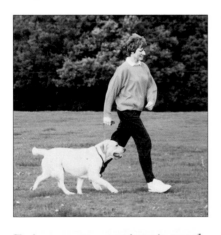

I N PART THREE, center stage belongs to you. You'll use your notebook to record personal data and write down your *insights* about the weighty matter of your relationship to food.

I hope you'll discover where your problems lie when you try to "Just say no" to the things that make you fat. Facing the dragons is the only way to slay them. We'll take a look at your *fitness* status. Being more active is truly the cornerstone of healthy weight loss. But there's no point in trying to become an athlete overnight. It simply won't work. Instead, I will guide you through a *self-assessment* of your individual state of fitness and make some suggestions for gradually increasing the amount of physical activity in your life. Then it will be time to set goals, both to motivate you and to help you measure your success.

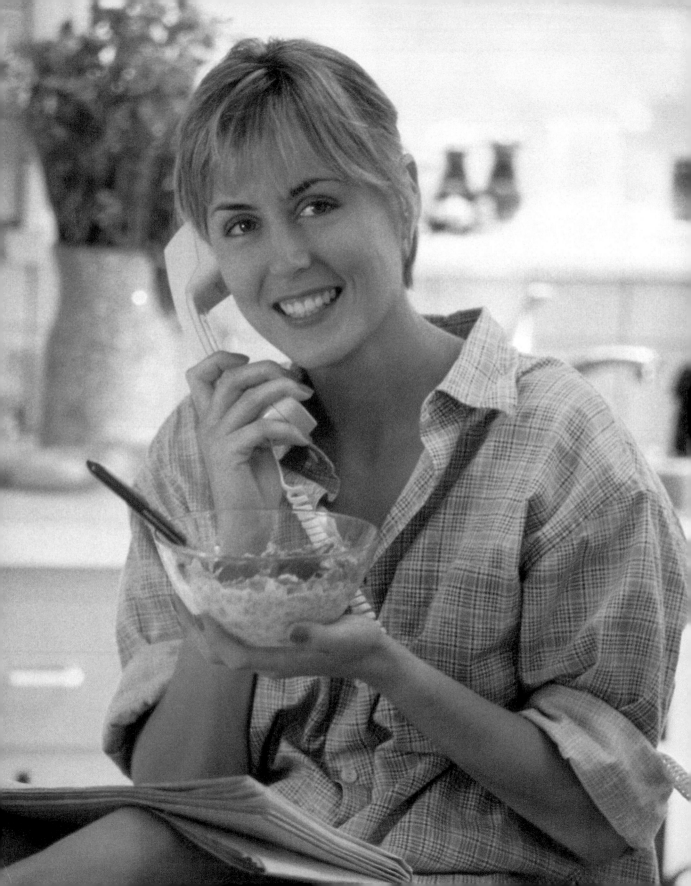

Chapter 7

What Does Food Mean to You?

Food, GLORIOUS FOOD! It is so much more than fuel to run our bodies. We all associate different things with foods, especially those foods we love. The goal of this chapter is to help you examine your personal eating psychology. Understanding what food means to you is the first step in modifying your behavior around food. And that, to put it simply, is the key to losing weight.

In this chapter...

✓ **Food as a symbol**

✓ **Understanding hunger triggers**

✓ **Emotional hunger**

✓ **Weight loss is about changing the way you behave**

✓ **Time to form a strategy**

✓ **Where will you go from here?**

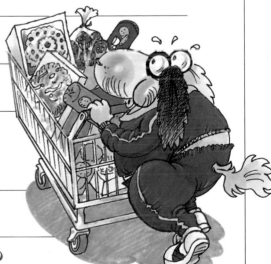

EATING WHILE READING OR TALKING ON THE TELEPHONE IS A HABIT TO BREAK

Food as a symbol

COMFORT FOOD: *A special treat as a reward for good behavior. Something sweet to console you when things aren't going your way. These are all non-nutritional uses of food. They are examples of food as a symbol. Think about the many associations you have with food. Delicious. Sensual. Refreshing. Piquant. Sweet. Nurturing. Festive. Sophisticated. Homey. Can you think of others?*

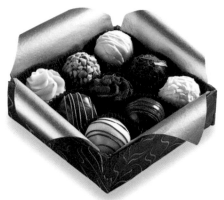

■ **Chocolates** *are a treat on special occasions and, given as gifts, are a symbol of love and affection.*

I'd be surprised if any of them had a thing to do with satisfying hunger or providing essential nutrients. If that was all that drove us to eat, losing weight would be a cinch and the Food Channel and a lot of cookbook publishers would be out of business. But the fact is, food has enormous emotional meaning. Eating often has nothing to do with physical hunger. Food choice only rarely is made on the basis of nutritional need.

Do not begin a diet or even try to adopt a more healthful approach to eating without recognizing what food means to you.

You will be pushing a huge rock up a steep mountain. And like Sisyphus in the Greek myth, the weight will come tumbling back on you time and time again.

FAT IS EVERYBODY'S ISSUE

Back in 1978, a therapist named Susie Orbach wrote *Fat Is a Feminist Issue*. This truly groundbreaking book is about weight loss, but it contains no diets. In essence, it is about the emotional weight that food, eating, and body image exerts on our lives. It is filled with valuable insights and helpful exercises (no, not the sweaty kind) you can use to gain a deeper understanding of what food and eating mean to you. It is still in print, and despite its title, I believe men could also benefit from many of the perceptions Orbach helps her readers gain about themselves.

Understanding hunger triggers

OVER THE COURSE *of an average day, your brain sends out many hunger messages. Often this is based on physiological fact: It's been about four hours since your last meal, and your stomach is empty. But at other times, something besides actual hunger has triggered the response.*

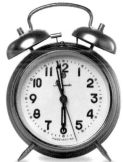

■ **Your body clock** *is set to expect food at certain times of the day, triggering hunger pangs.*

We all have habitual hunger buttons: We are used to eating at certain times of day, so that's when we "feel hungry." In addition to time of day, there are, for women especially, times of the month when eating is what we want to do. There are *physiological* reasons for this, most of them having to do with hormone levels.

Some drugs – prescription and recreational – push our hunger buttons. Others suppress hunger, and for that reason are used as "diet pills." In either case, alterations in brain chemistry are responsible for promoting or suppressing hunger. In addition, alcohol removes inhibitions, including, often, the resolve not to eat in excess of need.

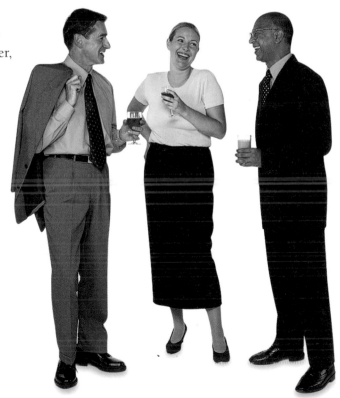

■ **Drinking alcohol** *often induces hunger, especially when consumed in excess. It can also lead to overeating.*

Even more triggers

There are places we associate with food and hunger. It may be our parents' home, our office, or a sporting event or movie theater. For me, the popcorn stand at the local multiplex is not a draw, but I am definitely in the minority. Think of places you visit regularly that make you want to chow down.

And of course, there are seasons in which we tend to eat more than usual. Many people consume more calories during the winter. There is a primitive and possibly physiological reason for this. Remember that one of the main functions of food is to provide the calories to maintain body heat. Especially if we live in cold climates and are often outdoors, we may feel a need to take in more calories. Although it is true that nowadays adequate clothing and well-heated indoor spaces take care of the problem, some instinct passed down by our cave-dwelling ancestors may trigger the desire for food.

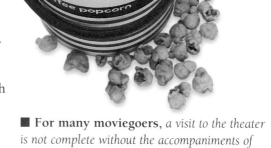

People can set off hunger alarms, too. These may be friends and colleagues with whom sharing a meal is a particular pleasure. Or it may be someone who inspires a negative response that makes us want to comfort ourselves with food.

■ **For many moviegoers,** *a visit to the theater is not complete without the accompaniments of popcorn and soft drinks.*

Certain occasions such as parties and other social gatherings are prime eating triggers. Anyone who has ever tried to squelch the urge to eat during a social occasion can attest to that. Smokers have a whole other set of triggers that can be particularly problematic.

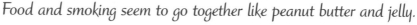

Food and smoking seem to go together like peanut butter and jelly.

Sometimes one is used as a substitute for the other, but more often they merely punctuate each other. Ending a meal with a cigarette may be increasingly difficult as more restaurants forbid the practice, but most smokers light up the minute they are outside. On the other side of the coin, smokers often resort to something flavorful to counteract the taste of their last puff.

Emotional hunger

WE ALSO HAVE EMOTIONAL HUNGER BUTTONS. Certain ways of feeling suggest food to us, either as a distraction from those emotions or as an accompaniment. For example, I feel the need to eat whenever I come home. It doesn't matter what time it is, or even how long it's been since I last ate. There's something about eating that says to me, "I'm home".

Many people eat when they're bored. Can you think of some emotional triggers that make you want to eat?

Depression and other mood triggers

Eating and depression often go hand in hand. There are many reasons for this. Psychologically, eating may be a way of seeking comfort when you are depressed. There are undoubtedly physiological influences as well, since certain chemicals in the brain are associated with both mood and hunger.

For some depressed people, engaging in behavior that makes them feel guilty is part of a cycle of depression. The worse they feel about themselves, the more they do things that make them feel bad about themselves.

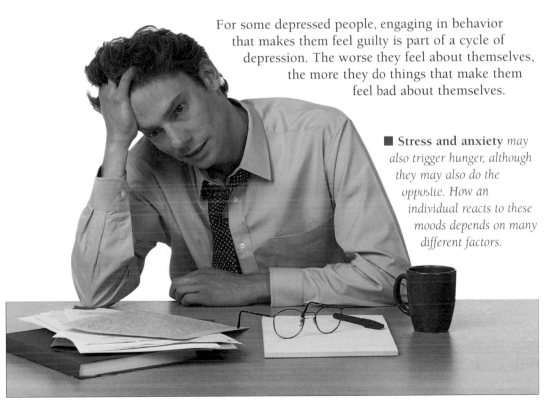

■ **Stress and anxiety** *may also trigger hunger, although they may also do the opposite. How an individual reacts to these moods depends on many different factors.*

Depression and anxiety are problems that should be discussed with and, if necessary, treated by a doctor.

If you think you are suffering from depression or anxiety, see a doctor as soon as possible. Do not begin a weight-loss effort without doing so.

If you do not discuss your worries with a doctor, not only will your efforts probably meet with failure, but yet another opportunity for self-blame may well worsen your mood problems.

EATING DISORDERS

These are very serious psychological problems. Bulimia and anorexia nervosa are the two best-known eating disorders. People suffering from anorexia nervosa starve themselves, sometimes literally to death. People with bulimia alternately gorge and purge, eating far in excess of normal and then vomiting to rid themselves of what they ate. Some people who suffer from eating disorders use laxatives and enemas to try to eliminate food from their system. All of these practices are dangerous to physical health. They are also symptoms of serious emotional disturbances in need of treatment.

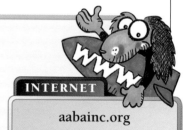

INTERNET

aabainc.org

The American Anorexia Bulimia Association offers information, support, and referral networks for people suffering from eating disorders.

Compulsive eating and bingeing are two other related eating disorders. If you eat when you are not really hungry and even though you know you should not, you are a compulsive eater. Compulsive eaters often eat for reasons that have nothing to do with hunger. Bingeing is a characteristic behavior of compulsive eaters, who in some cases may consume thousands of calories at a time. Unlike bulimics, they do not purge afterward. Most compulsive eaters are secretive about their eating habits and suffer from guilt and shame about the behavior.

One kind of compulsive eating is called night-eating syndrome (NES). People suffering from NES eat a lot at bedtime and even awaken during the night to eat. The result should not surprise you: weight gain, often to the point of obesity. Experts think there is a defect in these people's body clock.

Finally, diet addiction can be a sign of disordered eating. People who are constantly going on and off diets, continually losing and then regaining weight, may suffer from compulsive or other eating disorders.

Weight loss is about changing the way you behave

THE TROUBLE WITH MOST DIETS is that they call for a way
of eating that is virtually impossible to maintain for more than a short period
of time. To change your behavior you must be honest with yourself about what
you eat, how much you eat, when you eat, and most important, why you eat.

*The real secret to losing weight, and keeping it off, is changing
the way you behave around food.*

Many people insist they do not overeat. They talk about the modest meals
they eat, perhaps skipping breakfast in favor of a cup of black coffee. They
swear that lunch is just a salad or a diet shake. But somehow they forget to
mention – and probably have forgotten themselves – the midmorning muffin, that
handful of jelly beans
while chatting at a colleague's
desk, the Happy Hour free
hors d'oeuvres, a little taste
of this and sip of that while
preparing the family meal,
the bedtime snack.

Do you have similar "freelance"
eating episodes in your day?

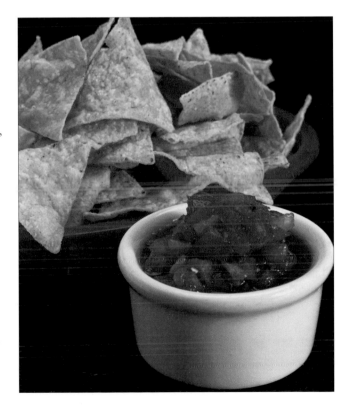

■ **When reviewing your eating
habits,** *it's easy to overlook those extra
snacks between meals such as that
bowl of tortilla chips you enjoyed with
predinner drinks.*

TEST YOURSELF

Here's a self-quiz to help you identify your own triggers. Take out your weight-loss notebook and start a new page with the heading "What Food Means to Me," and write your answers there. The answers to the quiz will provide knowledge that you can incorporate in the diet you ultimately design for yourself. For that reason, it is important that you be honest with yourself.

If you can't answer all the questions off the top of your head, observe your eating behavior over the course of a few days or a week, and add or revise your answers. Some questions require a calorie counter. Get one if you don't have one already. And pay particular attention to the true definition of a serving of everything you eat.

INTERNET

4weightloss.com

At this site you will find two very useful calorie guides: The Kitchen Counter and Fast Food Calculator.

1. How many meals do you eat in a typical day?

2. How many snacks do you eat in a typical day?

3. Do you ever eat when you are not hungry?

4. Do you ever eat at bedtime or during the night?

5. Do you ever eat alone?

6. How do you feel when you eat alone?

7. Do you eat different foods or quantities when you are alone than when you are with others?

8. When you cook or prepare food for yourself or others, do you taste and eat some of it during the preparation?

9. When you clean up and put or throw away uneaten food after a meal, do you eat some of it?

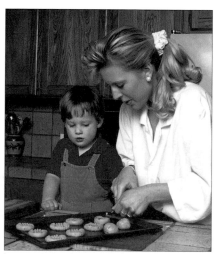

■ **When cooking or baking,** *how often do you have a nibble or a taste of the food while preparing it?*

10 What is/are your favorite food(s)?

11 What moods, feelings, or occasions inspire you to eat your favorite foods?

12 How often do you eat these foods?

13 What do you consider a "serving" of each of these foods (cups, ounces, pieces)?

14 How does this compare with the definition of a serving on the label?

15 How many calories are there in each serving?

16 How many calories are there in the amount you usually eat? (Multiply calories per serving by number of servings you eat.)

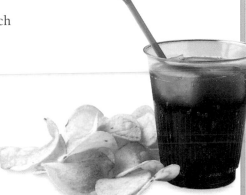

■ **Are there specific** *occasions that inspire you to go for junk food?*

17 What is your favorite beverage?

18 What moods, feelings, or occasions inspire you to drink it?

19 How often do you drink it?

20 What do you consider a "serving" of this beverage?

21 How does this compare with the definition of a serving on the label?

22 How many calories are there in each serving?

23 How many calories are there in the amount you usually drink? (Multiply calories per serving by number of servings you drink.)

24 What is your idea of comfort food?

25 What moods, feelings, or occasions inspire you to eat comfort food?

26 How often do you eat this food?

27 What do you consider a "serving" of this food (cups, ounces, pieces)?

28 How does this compare with the definition of a serving on the label?

29 How many calories are there in each serving?

30 How many calories are there in the amount you usually eat? (Multiply calories per serving by number of servings you eat.)

31 What food can't you stop eating once you begin?

32 What moods, feelings, or occasions inspire you to eat this food?

33 How often do you eat this food?

34 How much do you typically consume when you do eat this food?

35 How does this compare with the definition of a serving on the label?

36 How many calories are there in each serving?

37 How many calories are there in the amount you usually eat? (Multiply calories per serving by number of servings you eat.)

38 What do you consider a special occasion food or drink, to be consumed only infrequently?

39 According to what occasions, moods, or feelings do you consume this food or drink?

40 How often have you consumed it in the past month? Six months? Year?

41 How much do you typically consume on these occasions (cups, ounces, pieces)?

42 How does this compare with the definition of a serving on the label?

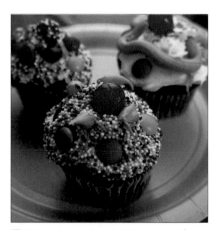

■ **Can you enjoy** *just one cupcake, or do you find it difficult to stop eating sweet foods once you start?*

43 How many calories are there in each serving?

44 How many calories are there in the amount you usually consume? (Multiply calories per serving by number of servings you eat.)

45 On what occasions do you find yourself eating more or less responsibly than you think you should?

46 In what places do you find yourself eating more or less responsibly than you think you should?

47 With which people do you find yourself eating more or less responsibly than you think you should?

48 At what times of day do you find yourself eating more or less responsibly than you think you should?

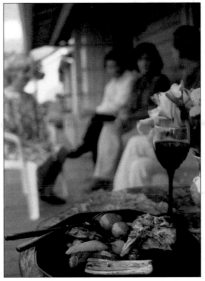

■ **Do you eat** *less responsibly when you are socializing with particular groups of people?*

49 On what days of the week do you find yourself eating more or less responsibly than you think you should?

50 At what times of the month do you find yourself eating more or less responsibly than you think you should?

51 At what times of the year do you find yourself eating more or less responsibly than you think you should?

52 Have you ever voluntarily vomited or taken laxatives or enemas to rid yourself of what you considered excess food?

53 Do you ever eat even when you are not hungry and when you know you shouldn't?

54 Do you ever eat huge amounts of a food, even when you are no longer hungry and know you should stop?

55 Do you ever eat when you are not hungry because you feel afraid that you will be hungry later?

56 What single word would you use to describe the mood around your family dinner table?

57 Was there a family rule about eating everything on your plate or otherwise not wasting food?

58 What was the attitude about second helpings at family meals in your childhood?

59 Is there anything about the way you eat or what you eat that resembles your childhood eating habits?

60 Is there anything about the way you eat or what you eat that is markedly different from your childhood eating habits?

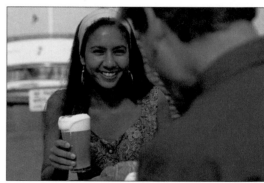

■ **How often do you** *eat or drink when you are not feeling particularly hungry?*

61 How many diets have you gone on in the past year?

62 What was the average duration of each one?

63 Was it longer or shorter than you originally planned?

64 Why did you stop eating according to the diet?

65 What was the purpose of the diet?

66 Did you achieve that goal?

ANALYZE YOUR ANSWERS

Take a look at your answers. Try to group them according to the following categories:

a **Normal eating behavior**

b **Dangerous or irresponsible eating behavior**

c **Childhood and family customs, behaviors, and attitudes**

d **Eating triggers:**
- Hunger
- Places
- Time of day
- People
- Day of week
- Occasions
- Time of month
- Moods
- Time of year
- Availability of specific foods

■ **Review your answers** *carefully: they will help you design a diet that works for you.*

e **Danger foods:**
- Foods or drinks I can't stop eating once I begin
- High-calorie or high-fat foods I eat often
- Foods I eat at night
- Foods I often eat as snacks
- Foods I eat more than one serving of at a time

f **Eating habits:**
- Habits and behaviors that help me eat responsibly
- Habits and behaviors that keep me from eating responsibly
- Habits and behaviors I think I can change
- Habits and behaviors that seem very difficult to change

Time to form a strategy

AFTER TAKING THE QUIZ and analyzing your answers, you should have a pretty good idea where food dangers lie for you. If you are like most people, you eat in response to triggers more often than in response to physiological hunger.

Knowing what your specific triggers are can help you modify your behavior in three different ways:

1. Avoid triggers: This may not always be possible, but it often will be. Take a look at your hunger triggers and see which ones you can avoid always or at least often. If family gatherings are nonstop food fests, perhaps you could suggest a noneating activity instead. If a jar of salted peanuts says "Eat all of me," ban peanuts from your home. If you eat less responsibly when you are alone, try to eat with others as often as possible.

2. Change the way you respond to triggers: When you cannot eliminate triggers from your life, you can substitute behavior. Instead of opening the refrigerator, how about opening a book and losing yourself in reading? Instead of walking to the cookie jar, how about taking a walk outside? Not only will that get you away from the cookie jar, it will burn some calories and maybe even lift the mood that made you want to reach for a sweet.

3. Find other ways to comfort yourself: When your mood makes you want comfort food, try a nonfood alternative. Perhaps a hot bath or a hug or sitting in a cozy chair with a blanket while listening to soothing music will answer your needs as well as a banana split or plate of meat loaf and mashed potatoes.

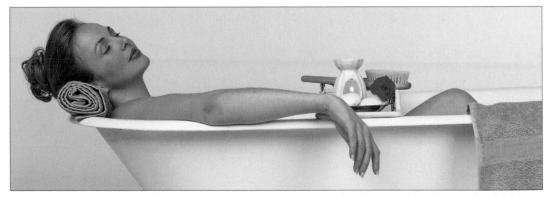

■ **Soothe away** *the cares of the day by relaxing in a hot bath rather than reaching for comfort foods. It's important to think of new ways to make yourself feel better and more positive about life.*

It's a fact of life that bad habits are easier to keep than good ones. Still, if you are able to identify things you do as habits, that's the first step in ridding yourself of the bad ones. I have suggested a few substitutions. Can you think of more that apply specifically to yourself and your circumstances?

It is difficult to just say no, but it is easier if you can replace one habit for another.

Make your own rules

Try to develop a set of rules for yourself. Write them down in your notebook and look at them frequently. Make a Food Blacklist: foods you simply do not eat. You'll be able to identify candidates for this list if you look at the answers to your quiz. Personally, roasted cashew nuts are my downfall. Once I eat one, I'll eat them all. I have made it a rule that I do not have them in the house. Because if I begin, I know I can easily consume my entire daily calorie requirement in one sitting and hate myself afterward.

A WRITING ASSIGNMENT

Take out your notebook and begin a new page. Your assignment is to write an essay on your hopes and fears about losing weight. It can be as long or as short as you like. It can even be a list. But think hard as you write and be sure to include everything you can think of on the subject. Explore your dreams about how you will look and feel, how your life will be different if you are able to lose some or all of your excess weight. Also think about how you will feel if you succeed in this challenge and if your success can be sustained over the long term.

Then think about what your fears are. Fear of failure is the most obvious, but you may also be afraid of success. Give that some thought. You may be afraid of your hunger, afraid you will not be able to handle situations that you have previously managed through eating. You may worry that you'll have to buy an entire new wardrobe or that your skin will sag. You may believe your mother or your spouse will still criticize your appearance or that even if you lose a good many pounds, you will still have curves where Kate Moss doesn't.

As with your personal database, this essay will be a valuable reference later on, when you are designing a weight-loss program that works for you, and after that, when you have made many of the changes you need to make to lead a healthier and more active life.

Where will you go from here?

BACK IN CHAPTER 1, *you took a hard look at your body and collected a lot of data to tell you whether you are overweight and, if so, by how much. In this chapter, I have asked you to think about your relationship to food and eating. Now it is time to decide whether you need to lose weight at all. And if you do, whether you are ready to make the commitment.*

I believe such a commitment is essential before you can make the changes in habit and behavior that are required for permanent weight loss.

Remember: We are not looking for a quick fix to lose weight. We are aiming for a change in lifestyle that is sustainable over the long term.

Losing a few pounds is simple; keeping them off is the goal. So, where will you go from here?

Knowing what's right for you

Perhaps you have discovered your weight is well within the normal range and your BMI is within the definition of healthy weight. You do not need to lose more weight, but I hope you will adopt or maintain an active lifestyle and the healthful eating habits we've been talking about. And if, over the course of time, your weight begins to creep into overweight territory, I hope you'll pick up this book again.

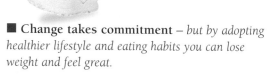

■ **Change takes commitment** – *but by adopting healthier lifestyle and eating habits you can lose weight and feel great.*

If your self-assessment tells you there's weight to be lost, but you are not ready to change your behavior and make a serious commitment to being more active and eating in a healthier way, it may make more sense to put the idea of weight loss on the back burner. Let it simmer, though, and revisit the idea from time to time. Perhaps talking to a doctor or friend will convince you that your health depends on it. Perhaps being more aware of your behavior around food and exercise will keep alive the thought of changing. Just because you aren't ready now doesn't mean you never will be.

But if you're ready to really do it, let's go full speed ahead!

A simple summary

✔ Food has symbolic meaning beyond its value as a nutritional substance needed for survival.

✔ Hunger is often a response to emotional triggers rather than physiological signals.

✔ Smokers often respond to hunger triggers dictated by their addiction to nicotine.

✔ Eating disorders are the result of chemical and emotional dysfunctions related to hunger triggers.

✔ Behavior modification is the key to weight loss.

✔ Understanding the meaning food has for you will help you modify your eating behavior.

✔ Making a Food Blacklist will help you avoid foods that you cannot eat responsibly.

✔ Commitment is essential to any successful weight-loss plan. Do not begin unless and until you are ready to commit to change.

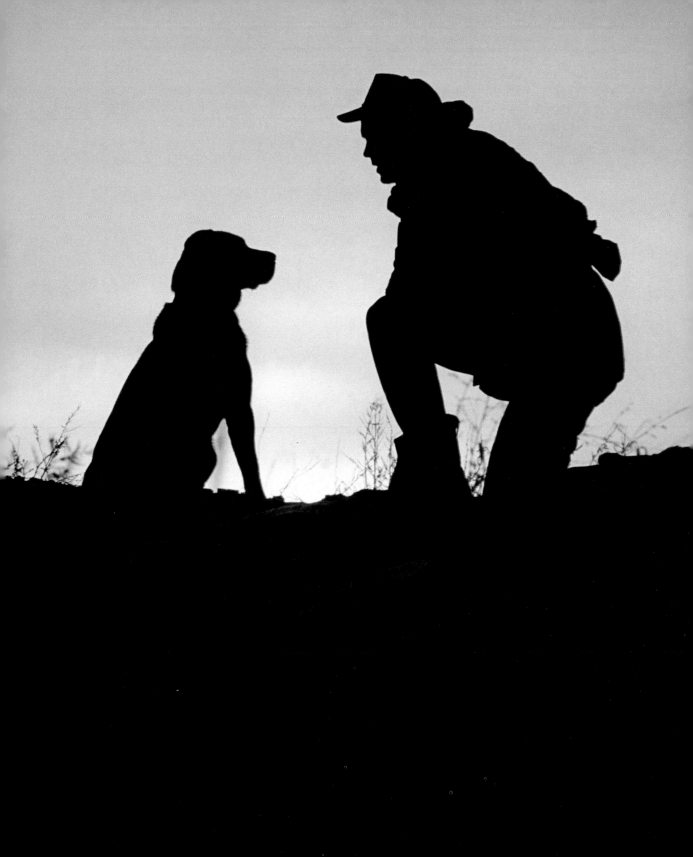

Chapter 8

How Fit Are You?

IF YOU WANT TO LOSE WEIGHT and keep it off, you cannot do it with diet alone. When it comes to being healthy, fitness is as important as normal weight. The next step on the road to weight loss is to take a good look at your current level of fitness and begin thinking about how you can be more active. Think of it as a preventive health checkup.

In this chapter...

✓ Is lack of stamina keeping you on the sidelines?

✓ A fitness review

✓ Your fitness scorecard

✓ Endurance

✓ Strength

✓ Flexibility

✓ Self-assessment

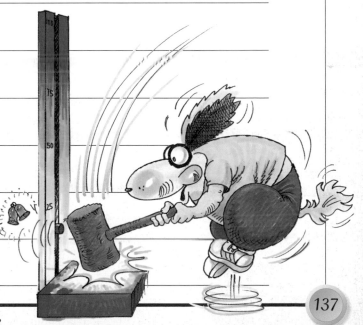

Is lack of stamina keeping you on the sidelines?

JUST AS YOU ROUND THE CORNER, *you see the bus pull into the bus stop. If you pick up your pace, you ought to make it before the last passenger gets on and the doors close. But by the time you get there, you're out of breath and your legs are aching, a sure sign that the muscles aren't getting enough oxygen. And the bus has pulled away. Oh well, by the time the next bus comes, the pain in your legs will have subsided and you ought to be breathing regularly.*

It's the company picnic and they're choosing up sides for volleyball. You know you should join in. Not only is it a chance for informal socializing with your supervisor and coworkers, but it's a great way to show the boss that you measure up as a team player, in more ways than one. But you also know you won't last 5 minutes, so you sit on the sidelines and hope you aren't losing too many "points."

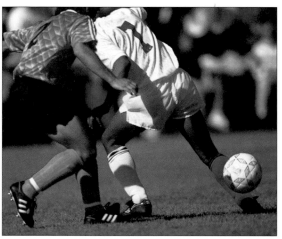

■ **Playing with a team** *requires stamina if you're not going to let down the side, so, if you're unfit, you probably won't want to participate in a group sport.*

It's a beautiful spring day and your 3- and 5-year-olds are playing tag. They call to you to join them, but after two times around the yard you've collapsed into a heap on the grass. "Come on," they urge, pulling at your arms, but when it's clear you're out of steam, they run off, dismissing you with "Aw, you're no fun." If you recognize yourself in any of these three scenarios, your problem is lack of *stamina.*

DEFINITION

The dictionary defines stamina *as vigor, endurance; the capacity to withstand fatigue or disease. Plain and simple, it's your "get up and go," and what makes it possible for you to keep on going. Stamina is an important sign of fitness and health.*

A fitness review

TO RECAP *what we learned in Chapter 3, the components of fitness are endurance, strength, and flexibility.*

INTERNET

www.shapeup.org/ fitness

This section of the ShapeUp America! web site begins with a "Physical Activity Readiness Questionnaire" (PAR-Q) to help you determine whether it is safe to begin to be more active. Other features include a fitness test and suggestions for appropriate activities for each level of fitness.

Your endurance is largely determined by your cardiorespiratory health. If you are overweight and generally inactive, your heart and lungs have to work overtime to keep oxygenated blood circulating throughout your body.

Your strength is largely determined by the condition of your muscles, whereas your flexibility depends on joints and connective tissues (ligaments and tendons) as well as muscles. Again, overweight and inactivity have a negative effect on both strength and flexibility.

Being fit is like money in the bank, but you have to keep up your deposits.

Regular moderate activity will help you maintain fitness.

The more active you are, the more fit you are likely to be and to remain as you grow older.

■ **Flexibility is key** *to fitness. If you can turn at the waist and see what's behind you, that's a good indicator of flexibility. If you can't, consider embarking on a program to help get you into better physical shape.*

Your fitness scorecard

TAKE OUT YOUR WEIGHT-LOSS NOTEBOOK. *We'll be doing some tests, so keeping a record of your answers will help you see where you started and how far you've traveled on your journey to your weight and fitness goals.*

Date	10/1			
My resting heart rate (RHR)	80			
My maximum heart rate (MHR)	185			
My target heart rate (THR) 60%/80%	114 / 148			
My basal metabolic rate (BMR)	2,000			
My daily calorie needs to maintain weight	2,400			
My daily calorie goal to lose weight	1,900			

MY FITNESS FACTS

Lifestyle/activity score	2			
Endurance:				
Number of jumping jacks	15			
Pulse	180			
Time to RHR	3 mins			
Strength:				
Number of chest lifts	10			
Flexibility:				
Inches reached	25 in			

■ **Record your fitness facts** *so you can review them as part of your fitness program. With regular exercise, you should notice a difference within weeks.*

Endurance

YOUR HEARTBEAT IS AN IMPORTANT GAUGE *of cardiorespiratory fitness. Significant variables are how fast it beats when you are doing nothing and when you are exercising, and how quickly it returns to the resting state after you have stopped. Your heart rate, or pulse, is measured as beats per minute. Each beat represents a contraction of the heart muscle as it pumps out blood.*

Resting heart rate

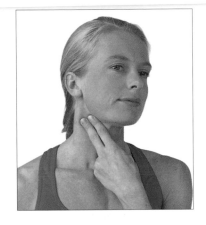

At rest, the typical number of heartbeats per minute is 70. This figure, known as the resting heart rate (RHR), varies from person to person with the normal range between 60 and 100 beats per minute. In general, the slower the resting heartbeat within the normal range, the better.

What's your normal resting heart rate? Here's a simple way to find out. Do this when you haven't been exercising or exerting yourself in any other way. You'll need a watch or clock with a second hand.

1. Find a pulse. The easiest ones to locate are on either side of your neck just below your jawbone or on the underside of either wrist.

2. Firmly but gently place your index and middle fingers on one of these points. (Don't use your thumb. It has its own pulse, which will confuse matters.)

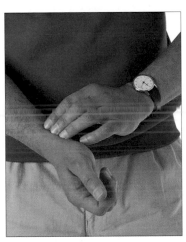

3. Once you feel the pulse strongly, count the beats for 15 seconds.

4. Multiply the number of beats by 4 to get your resting heart rate.

5. Try it a few times over the course of one or more days and average out your results.

6. Enter your RHR into your personal database.

■ **Take your pulse** *for 15 seconds, and multiply the number of beats by 4. For example: 20 beats per 15 seconds x 4 = 80 beats per minute, which is your RHR.*

Maximum heart rate

Maximum heart rate, or MHR, is the theoretical highest number of times per minute the human heart can beat. Only in times of extreme stress will your heart beat that fast. MHR varies considerably from person to person, but in general, it decreases with age.

You can figure your MHR by subtracting your age from the number 220. For example, if you are 35 years old, your MHR would be 185.

Fear, stress, and anxiety can raise your heartbeat, as can some serious health conditions. An increased heartbeat may be an appropriate temporary response to a stressful situation or it may be a cause for concern.

It is never a good idea to exert yourself to the point of MHR.

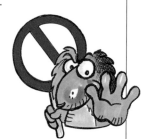

Target heart rate

If your resting heart rate is at one end of the scale and your maximum heart rate is at the other, your *target heart rate* (THR) occupies a range between them.

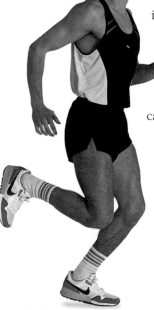

When you exert yourself physically, your heart beats faster than when you are at rest. Exercise causes a temporary increase in your heart rate, and that is a good thing. In fact, it is one of the goals of physical activity. When you exercise, you should aim for the THR range appropriate for your age (see chart opposite).

Aerobic exercise is considered the ideal way to achieve cardiovascular fitness.

In general, effective aerobic activity consists of 20 to 30 minutes of exertion at an intensity that raises the heartbeat to 60 to 80 percent of the maximum heart rate (MHR).

So the target heart rate for aerobic conditioning is between 60 and 80 percent of your MHR. The American Heart Association recommends a slightly lower target range for optimal fitness of 50 to 75 percent.

■ **Running** *is a good way of improving your cardiovascular fitness.*

For example, say you are 35 years old. Your MHR is 185 (220-35). Sixty percent of that is 111; 80 percent is 148. An aerobic workout

TARGET HEART RATE

AGE	MHR	50%	60%	75%	80%
20	200	100	120	150	160
25	195	98	117	146	156
30	190	95	114	143	152
35	185	93	111	139	148
40	180	90	108	135	144
45	175	88	105	131	110
50	170	85	102	128	136
55	165	83	99	124	132
60	160	80	96	120	128
65	155	78	93	116	124
70	150	75	90	113	116
75	145	73	87	109	116
80	140	70	84	105	112

Calculating your MHR and THR zone

$$220 - your\ age\ \underline{\quad} = MHR\ \underline{\quad}$$

$$your\ MHR\ \underline{\quad}\ x\ .60 = lower\ limit\ \underline{\quad}$$

$$your\ MHR\ \underline{\quad}\ x\ .80 = upper\ limit\ \underline{\quad}$$

$$THR\ zone = \underline{\quad}\ to\ \underline{\quad}$$

■ **Work out your maximum heart rate** *and target heart rate zone, then record these on the fitness scorecard in your personal database.*

for you would involve getting your heart rate to between 111 and 148 beats per minute, and keeping it there for 20 to 30 minutes. Using the American Heart Association recommendation, you would aim to keep your heart rate between 95 and 139 beats per minute.

Another gauge of fitness is how long it takes or how hard you have to work to get to your target heart rate. It may seem backward, but the fact is a sedentary person who is relatively unfit will get to the target rate sooner and stay there longer than a fit person engaging in the same activity. Think of it this way: You and your friend, the superjock, are out for a run. After a quarter mile, whose heart is pounding to beat the band? And which one of you has to rest for 15 minutes before you can make it up the front steps?

It's very good to get your heart beating fast periodically, but you wouldn't want it racing all the time.

The faster your heart returns from the neighborhood of its MHR to its RHR, the fitter you are.

If all this pulse taking and mathematics seem too complicated for you, here's a simpler way to monitor the intensity of your workout:

■ **Can you walk and talk?** If you can keep up a conversation while walking or engaging in another physical activity, you are not working too hard.

■ **Oh, say can you sing?** If you can sing without slackening your level of effort, you are not working hard enough.

■ **Breathless?** If all you can do is gasp for breath, you are exercising too intensely.

If you haven't exercised in a long time, or at all, don't aim for your highest target heart rate.

As with any physical activity, you should start slowly and work your way up to your peak. Begin at the lower end of your target zone and maintain that level for a week or more. Then gradually work your way up, building the intensity of your activities until you reach the upper limit. If you want to challenge yourself further, you can try to push the limit, but never exceed 85 percent of your MHR.

If you are extremely overweight, over 60 years of age, take blood pressure medication, or suffer from a chronic disease or disabling condition, don't engage in any new physical activity without checking with your doctor.

■ **When you start to exercise,** *build up your activity level gradually. Begin at the lower end of your target zone and work your way up steadily.*

INTERNET

www.americanheart.org

If you want to know more about your heart and how to keep it healthy, log on to the American Heart Association web site. You'll find tips for heart-safe exercising for all ages and an interactive risk assessment of your personal heart health.

Strength

THERE ARE MORE THAN 650 MUSCLES *in your body. Some are stronger than others. Many fitness assessments ask how many push-ups or sit-ups you can do, on the assumption that upper arm and abdominal strength reflect the general state of your muscular fitness. This may or may not be true, depending on your age and whether you have a disability that affects only part of your body.*

Here are some general principles regarding muscular strength:

a Strength is dependent on both muscle mass and tone.

b Muscle mass and tone can be increased through weight-bearing exercise.

c Because muscle mass is dependent on testosterone, men have more massive muscles than women.

d Muscle mass and tone increase throughout adolescence and then begin to decline with age. Testosterone levels are the main reason for this.

e The greater the muscle mass, the greater the energy demand and the higher the metabolic rate, which is why more muscular people require more calories to maintain bodily functions.

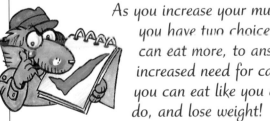

As you increase your muscle mass, you have two choices. You can eat more, to answer the increased need for calories. Or you can eat like you always do, and lose weight!

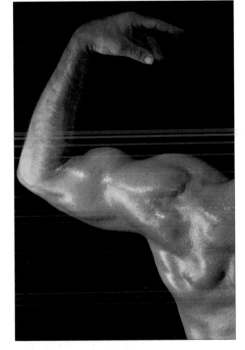

■ **Men are more muscular** *than women because muscle mass is dependent on levels of testosterone, which is present in women only in small amounts.*

145

Flexibility

FLEXIBILITY IS A REFLECTION *of how well your muscles, joints, ligaments, and tendons can stretch and bend. When you bend over at the waist with arms outstretched, how close to do you come to touching your toes? Your ankles? Your knees? Can you turn at the waist and see what's behind you? Can you reach over the top of your head and touch your opposite ear? These are all indicators of flexibility.*

Your flexibility probably varies throughout the day. We are all stiffer in the morning, after a night's rest, and become more flexible as we "warm up" through normal activity during the day. If you lead a sedentary life, multiply that morning effect by years and you will get an idea of how habitual inactivity affects flexibility. And it will only get worse with age.

If you do not want to be a stooped old person for whom rising from a chair is agony, focus on flexibility as you aim to get fit.

Self-assessment

THERE ARE MANY FITNESS TESTS OUT THERE, *most of which require you to exert yourself in various ways and observe the results in terms of the three components of fitness. Thanks to the wealth of fitness and weight-loss sites on the Internet, you can find one version or another of these tests online. You may want to try them. If you do, print out the results and put them in your weight-loss notebook.*

INTERNET

www.phys.com/fitness/ analysis

This is one of many sites with a fitness test you can perform at home. It will evaluate your results and give you a personal fitness score.

What follows is a much simpler self-assessment. I also think it's a more effective one because you are measuring yourself against yourself rather than against some theoretically fit person you've never met! It consists of a brief quiz about your level of physical activity and three fitness yardsticks.

Keep a record of this self-assessment in your notebook and look at it periodically, say once a month, as you gradually become more active. The improvement you see will be one of the best motivators to keep up your personal program. The yardsticks require you to exert yourself physically.

Even though they are relatively mild, don't try the physical yardstick tests without consulting your doctor if you have heart problems, are taking blood pressure medication, or have arthritis.

LIFESTYLE ACTIVITY QUIZ

Your lifestyle is a pretty good indication of your fitness. Imagine a scale that runs from sedentary through somewhat active and moderately active to very active. Take this brief quiz on your exercise habits to give you an idea where you fall on the fitness spectrum.

1 Do you engage in regularly scheduled exercise?
No (0 points) ❏ **Yes** (1 point) ❏

2 If so, how long is each exercise session?
15 minutes (1 point) ❏ **30 minutes** (2 points) ❏ **45 minutes** (3 points) ❏
An hour (4 points) ❏ **More than an hour** (5 points) ❏

3 How many times a week?
1 (1 point) ❏ **2** (2 points) ❏ **3** (3 points) ❏ **4** (4 points) ❏
5 (5 points) ❏ **6** (6 points) ❏ **7** (7 points) ❏

4 Do you exert yourself physically during the course of normal activities at work or around the house?
No (0 points) ❏ **Yes** (1 point) ❏

Add up the numbers given after each choice.

Your score:	Your lifestyle:
■ 0–3 points	Sedentary
■ 4–5 points	Somewhat active
■ 6–8 points	Moderately active
■ 9 points or more	Very active

A simple measure of your endurance

Wearing a comfortable pair of sports shoes that give you support, do as many jumping jacks as you can before you feel out of breath. Count out loud as you jump. Immediately take your pulse for 15 seconds, then write down the number of jumping jacks you did and your pulse rate multiplied by 4. Note also if the resulting heart rate is higher or lower than your THR zone.

A minute after you stop jumping, take your pulse again for 15 seconds. Continue taking your pulse every minute until it returns to your resting heart rate.

JUMPING JACKS

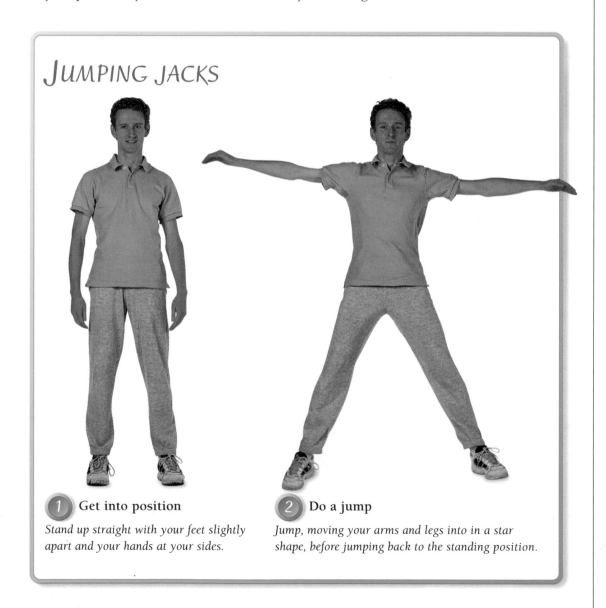

1 **Get into position**

Stand up straight with your feet slightly apart and your hands at your sides.

2 **Do a jump**

Jump, moving your arms and legs into in a star shape, before jumping back to the standing position.

Once you start exercising regularly, do this test once a month. If 15 jumping jacks got you to your THR the first time, could you do 20 a month later? If it took 3 minutes to return to your RHR the first time, did it take less time a month later? These are signs that your cardiovascular fitness is improving.

A simple measure of your strength

Strong abdominal muscles are only part of the strength picture, but they are important ones. Not only do they look good in a bathing suit, but also they help support your body, taking stress off your back.

Many back problems can be traced to flabby abdominal muscles.

To measure your strength, see how many chest lifts you can do. Concentrate on maintaining the proper form and do not pull at your neck or use your back muscles during any part of the exercise. Write down how many perfect chest lifts you did. Then test yourself again a month later. Will you be able to do five more? Ten? This is an indication that your abdominal muscle strength has increased.

CHEST LIFTS

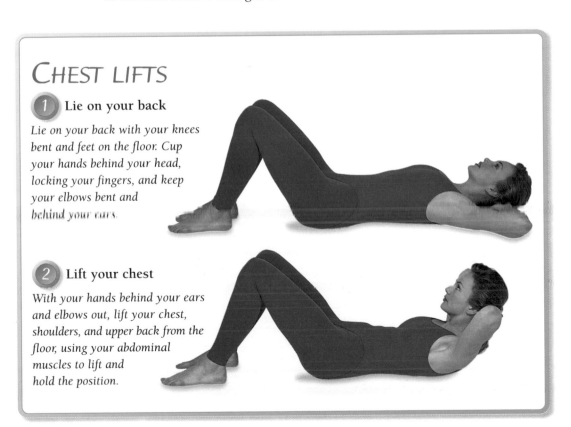

1 Lie on your back

Lie on your back with your knees bent and feet on the floor. Cup your hands behind your head, locking your fingers, and keep your elbows bent and behind your ears.

2 Lift your chest

With your hands behind your ears and elbows out, lift your chest, shoulders, and upper back from the floor, using your abdominal muscles to lift and hold the position.

A simple measure of your flexibility

Sit on the floor with your legs outstretched, feet flexed. That is, your toes should be pointed to the ceiling. Place a tape measure or yardstick along the side of your legs, with the beginning at your buttocks. Inhale, and as you exhale, stretch your hands forward as you bend at the waist. When you have reached as far as you can, look at the measure.

How many inches did you reach? Write this down in your notebook. Then try again a month later. Will you be able to increase your reach by an inch? Two inches? More? This is an indication that your flexibility has increased.

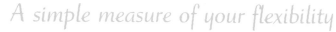

Keep your knees straight

Keep your toes pointed to the ceiling

Place a tape measure or yardstick beside you, beginning at your buttocks and ending at your heel, to see how far you can reach

■ **From this sitting position** *stretch your hands forward as you bend at the waist. How far can you reach? This is a measure of your flexibility.*

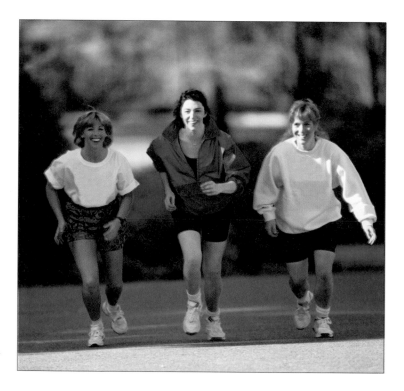

■ **The same active lifestyle** *that improves your fitness will also help you lose weight and maintain that loss. It will also be fun!*

Get the picture

Although it is entirely possible that you are as fit as a fiddle, chances are there's room for improvement in all the measures of fitness. You may be most interested in losing weight, but increasing your endurance, strength, and flexibility will pay more dividends because it will help you keep the weight off in the long term.

A simple summary

✓ Improving your fitness is the most effective route to permanent weight loss.

✓ Fitness is a combination of endurance, strength, and flexibility.

✓ Effective exercise should raise your heart rate to a target range within 50 to 80 percent of your maximum heart rate.

✓ Exercising 20 to 30 minutes at your target heart rate will increase your endurance.

✓ Increasing muscle mass increases your daily calorie needs and speeds your metabolism.

✓ Strengthening your abdominal muscles will improve your appearance and take stress off your back.

✓ Increasing and maintaining your flexibility will have lifelong benefits.

✓ If you have been inactive or suffer from health problems, consult your doctor before doing physical self-assessment or increasing activity.

✓ Measuring your own baseline level of fitness and retesting yourself periodically is a good way to monitor the effectiveness of your exercise program.

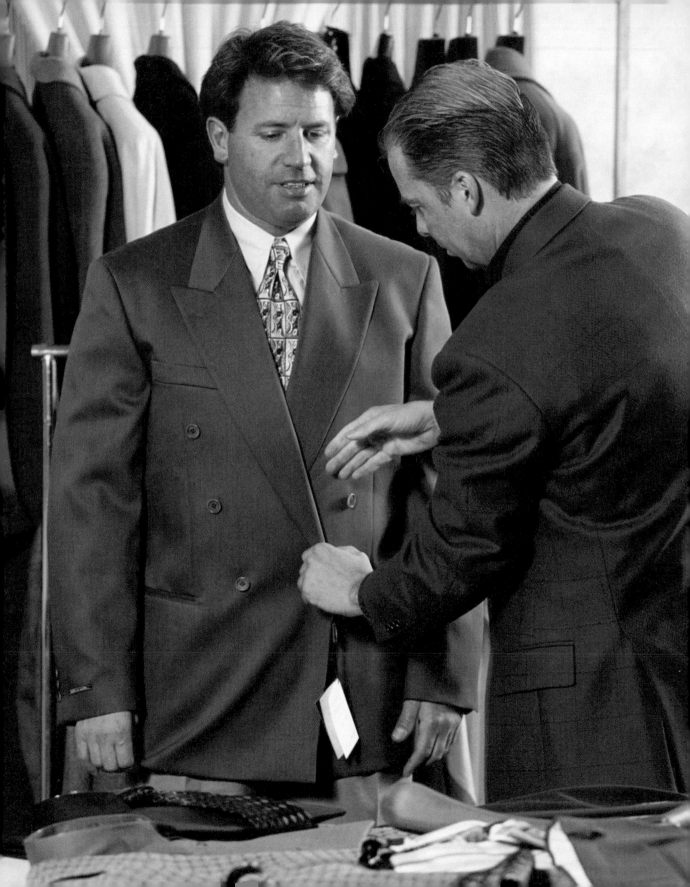

Chapter 9

Setting Goals

LOSING WEIGHT IS A LOT LIKE ROCK CLIMBING. For some it might be like conquering Everest, for others it's more like climbing the foothills. But it's never a walk in the woods. Let's take a look now at the size of the rock you'll be climbing and then set some goals. How far is the summit, and do you want to reach it? How fast will you climb? Will you do it in stages? What aids will you use? Will you do it alone or with a team?

In this chapter...

✓ Observe yourself

✓ Keeping focused

✓ Your weight-loss goals

✓ Your fitness goals

✓ Your plan

✓ Making a contract

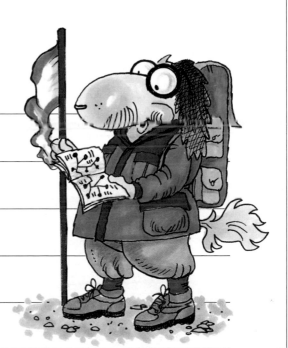

MEASURING UP FOR A SMALLER SUIT SIZE COULD BE A SHORT- OR LONG-TERM GOAL

Observe yourself

BEFORE YOU CAN BEGIN TO SET GOALS, *you need to take a long hard look at where you are now. Keeping a food and activity diary is the best way to do this. If you look at the times of day or moods you're in when you exercise and eat, you may even get ideas about substituting one for the other. (Guess which one?)*

It may seem like a bother, but keeping a diary will force you to see where your problems lie. Do yourself a favor and do it for a week. This diary is for you and you alone. No one else will read it.

When keeping your food diary you must promise to be honest with yourself.

Your diary should be kept in your weight-loss notebook, but if the notebook is too big to carry around, slip some index cards in your pocket or purse to note what you eat and how long you do what kind of exercise when you're away from home. You can enter this data in your notebook at the end of the day.

Your food diary

This will be an important tool for the eating side of your weight-loss plan. Combined with your answers to the quiz in Chapter 7 about what food means to you, the food diary will show you, in black and white, why you are overweight and what eating and behavior habits you need to change. You may be surprised how much food you consume in a typical day.

You may notice that certain moods, people, or circumstances accompany pig-outs.

You may spot dangerous times of day or a pattern of increased eating as the day progresses. Weekends may be perilous, or maybe business lunches are your undoing.

INTERNET

www.4weightloss.com

Click on Keeping Track and you'll find links to several calorie counters and activity calculators.

You will need to fill in the number of calories of everything you eat. If what you eat comes in a package, you can get this information from the label. (Remember: 10 cookies is not a serving!) Otherwise, use a calorie-counting book or one of the online calorie counters.

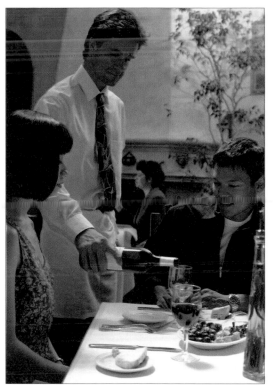

■ **When eating in a restaurant,** *make a rough estimate of the amounts of food consumed and don't forget to take drinks, including wine, into account.*

Don't get hung up on details. If aren't sure about quantities, estimate. But estimate on the high side.

A sample food diary can be found on the next page. Set up something similar in your weight-loss notebook, so that you have a food diary for each day of the week. On the page for the last day of the week, make a space for your weekly calorie total.

Set aside a column or space each day for comments. Use this space to write anything that will help you understand what was going on when you ate, including triggers or moods, anything about the occasion or people you were with, feelings of guilt or triumph you experienced before, during, or afterward.

As part of your food diary, record how many glasses of water you drink. Aim for a minimum of eight glasses or 64 ounces of water each day.

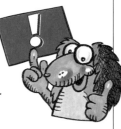

It's important to keep track of how much water you drink to remind you to drink a lot of it. Monitor your water consumption by making a check mark for each 8-ounce glass you drink. It's easiest if you measure out your water in advance, but if you drink from a water fountain, for example, you can figure two swallows per ounce.

■ **Water contains** *no calories, so there's no counting there – but what you do have to keep track of is whether you're drinking enough of it.*

Daily food diary

Day MONDA
BREAKFAST 7
FOOD
Coffee
1/2&1/2
Toast
Butter
Jam
OJ
Calorie tota

COMMENTS
Usual bre

LUNCH Tin
FOOD
Bacon che
Large fries
Chocolate

Calorie to

COMMEI
I wa

Daily food diary

Day MONDAY   Date   12/6

DINNER Time 8 pm

FOOD	SERVINGS	CALORIES
Pizza	3 slices	690
Diet cola	12 oz	0
Calorie total:		690

COMMENTS (hunger level, place, people, etc.)

Exhausted when I got home, in no mood to cook

SNACKS

TIME	FOOD	SERVINGS	CALORIES
11 am	Glazed donut	1	250
	Coffee	1	5
	1/2 & 1/2	1 tbs	20
5 pm	Chocolate bar / 2 oz	1	300
7 pm	Beer / 12 oz	2	280
11 pm	2% milk	8 oz	120
	Oatmeal cookies	6	570
	Calorie total:		1,545

COMMENTS (hunger level, place, people, etc.)

Needed the energy boost at 5 and the beers later after the day I had

Water: (Check each 8 oz. glass) ☑ ☑ ☑ ☑ ☑ ☑ ○ ○

Total calories: 4,122

■ **This is just a made-up food diary,** *but have you ever had a day like this? Are you surprised how many calories this person managed to pack in? Can you identify the triggers? Can you point out the bad habits? Can you think of alternatives that could cut the calorie total? Did this person drink enough water?*

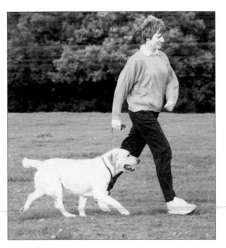

Your activity diary

When it comes to activity, be sure to enter things you do as a matter of routine (such as walking the dog or playing catch with your kids) as well as planned exercise. You may be pleasantly surprised to see how much motion there is in your day. On the other hand, you may see that most of your activity takes place on weekends. You may see slots on other days where you could fit in some more activity.

To get a full picture of your daily calorie burn, add your BMR (basal metabolic rate) to the number of calories burned by activities.

■ **Whatever type of exercise** *you do during the day, even if it's taking the dog for a walk in the local park, make sure you record it in your activity diary.*

See Chapter 5, page 94, to figure out what your BMR is.

A sample activity diary can be found on the next page. Make one like this in your weight-loss notebook for the entire week. Leave space on the last day for your total weekly calorie expenditure. In our sample, the number of calories burned for each exercise session assumes that the diarist is a somewhat active 160-pound male. To find the number of calories you have burned in a given activity, use one of the online activity calculators, or "burn barometers." As with your food diary, there is space to write your comments. Write in anything that will give you clues about how and where to fit activity into your day.

a. Were you tired when you began, but more energetic afterward? Maybe exercising after work is a way to add hours to your day.

b. Did you burn more calories when you exercised with a friend or went to a class than you did when you worked out alone?

c. Are you more likely to exercise at home or as part of some organized activity? Try to plan your exercise to take advantage of this.

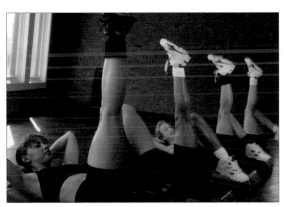

■ **Look for patterns** *in your diary. If, for example, you burn more calories in a class than when exercising alone, being an exercise groupie may be the way to go.*

Activity diary

Day   MONDAY   Date   9/1

Activity	Time	Duration	Calories burned	Place	Comments (mood, place, people, etc.)
Walked dog	7 a.m.	15 mins	72	Around block	Rain made it quick
Bike ride	5.30 p.m.	30 mins	217	Park	Slowish with kids
Yoga class	8 p.m.	60 mins	290	Y	Felt great after class

NOTES
Total calories burned: 579
BMR: 11 x 160 = 1,760 + 528 (30% of 1,760) = 2,288
Total daily calorie expenditure: 2,867

Day   Date

Activity	Time	Duration	Calories burned	Place	Comments (mood, place, people, etc.)

NOTES

■ **This activity diary** *was compiled by a fictional, somewhat active 160-pound male. His total daily calorie expenditure is 2,867, which means that if he consumes no more calories than this on a daily basis and maintains the same level of activity, he shouldn't gain weight.*

Keeping focused

A CASUAL INTENTION to eat more wisely, exercise more frequently, and drop some pounds is unlikely to be successful. Nor is promising yourself that you'll lose 10 pounds, by hook or by crook, in time for next month's high school reunion. You need a plan and the firm resolve to follow it. It has to be realistic. Like it or not, 10 pounds in a month is not realistic unless you're willing to gain it all back.

The best way to stay focused is to set both short- and long-term goals.

When you set short- and long-term goals, a single failure to reach a short-term goal is far less discouraging. You can revise your plan without throwing it all out the window. And when you succeed in reaching one of your milestones, you will feel all the more motivated to keep going to the next one.

Be realistic

A realistic short-term goal is to add 15 minutes of exercise to your day. Another one might be to ban snacking between dinner and bedtime. If you have been gaining weight, a reasonable short-term goal is to stop that gain in its tracks.

If you want (or need) to lose a specific number of pounds, you also want to be sure to keep them off. Depending on how much you plan to lose, stretch that loss over 6 months to a year. That's your long-term goal.

You will probably shed the first few pounds quickly, and then see a slowdown as you reach a weight-loss plateau.

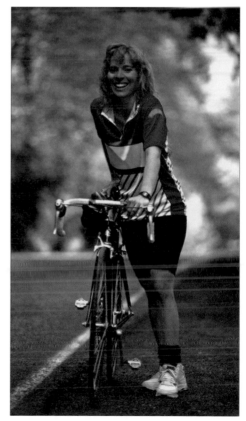

■ **Decide on a goal** *that is achievable for the next couple of weeks, or month, such as going for a 15-minute bike ride when you get home from work.*

We've spoken about the reasons for the plateau and what to do about it, and you'll find some strategies for moving beyond the plateau in Chapter 18. For now, you should build the plateau into your expectations.

If you want to lose 10 pounds over 6 months, for example, you might set a goal of a pound a week for the first month and then a pound every 2 weeks for the next two months. In the last 3 months the remaining 2 pounds will come off slowly and you will be concentrating on weight maintenance and solidifying your modified behavior. These are all short-term goals.

It would be realistic to try a similar pattern with 20 pounds, but to lose more than that you should take at least a year. If this sounds slow, it is.

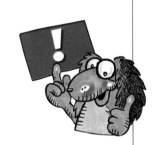

I cannot emphasize strongly enough that quick weight loss leads to quicker weight gain.

It takes time to replace bad habits with good ones. Fad diets tinker with your body chemistry. Highly restricted diets are short-term solutions to a long-term problem. You cannot sustain these diets over the long haul.

■ **Adopting a healthier**
lifestyle will bring lasting benefits and do far more good than fad diets, which are just temporary solutions.

Eating sensibly and exercising regularly are lifetime decisions. And their benefits are long lasting.

Your weight-loss goals

I KNOW I SOUND LIKE A BROKEN RECORD when I talk about the benefits of exercise and the primary importance of fitness. You bought this book because you want to lose weight. So humor me and I'll humor you. It's a win-win situation. But we'll begin with your weight-loss goals.

Where are you now?

Take a look at your personal database. If you haven't weighed yourself for a while, do it now and, if necessary, change your current weight and write in today's date. Has your weight changed since your last weighing session? Is it higher? Lower? Do you know why?

MEET JANE DOE

Jane Doe is 5 ft 4 in tall and weighs 150 pounds. According to the USDA height-weight table, she is moderately overweight. According to the BMI table, she is a 26, also moderately overweight. The healthy weight range for her height is between about 115 and 145. To get her BMI to 24, she'll have to lose 10 pounds.

How much she wants to lose is more complex. Does she want to be at the low end of her healthy weight or the high end or somewhere in the middle? Does she want to just edge in on a BMI of 24 or does she want to aim for 21 or 22? Does she want to climb Mount Everest or just that nice hill from which she can see a good sunset?

Jane decides on a middle range. She'd like to lose 20 pounds, giving her a BMI of 22 and a long-term goal of 130 pounds.

Where do you want to go?

Now take a look at your ideal weight. You can use the weight range from the height–weight table, but I recommend basing this figure on a combination of your BMI and the height-weight range. Take a look at the BMI and height-weight range charts on pages 25 and 32 and see how far you are from a healthy weight. Then consider carefully how much of a climb you want to make.

How long will you take?

The next thing to do is to break up your journey into bite-size pieces. Don't try to lose 10, 20, or more pounds as soon as you possibly can. That's not a rational plan. It won't keep you focused on the goal and it won't provide you feedback – encouraging or discouraging – on how you're doing. Now you can start to work out a plan for yourself. Be sure it incorporates a realistic view of what's happening in your personal life in the months ahead. Are there any predictable pitfalls in your timetable? If so, revise it to take them into account. If you need inspiration, read on to see how Jane Doe planned her timetable.

■ **Set up your own timetable** *on a new page in your notebook, sketching out a plan that you know is realistic for you.*

WHAT JANE PLANNED

It's mid-September and Jane's just had a lousy summer. The beach was out of the question, given what she looks like in a bathing suit, and her thighs chafed terribly in the hot weather. She'd like to be able to wear one of those lovely sleeveless cotton dresses come next June, but she knows several pig-out winter holidays lie between now and strawberry season. Here's the weight-loss timetable she designed for herself:

LONG-TERM GOAL: Lose 20 pounds in 9 months

Milestones: October 1–October 31 Lose 1 pound a week, for a total of 4 pounds

○ Goal weight on November 1: 146

Comment: Will probably be easy and a good motivator

Milestones: November 1–November 30 Lose 4 more pounds, for a total of 8 pounds

○ Goal weight on December 1: 142

Comment: Thanksgiving may spell D-A-N-G-E-R

Milestones: December 1–December 31 Maintain new weight through holidays

Comment: Keep away from the eggnog!

Milestones: January 1–January 31 Lose 4 more pounds, for a total of 12 pounds

○ Goal weight on February 1: 138

Comment: Make a New Year's Resolution

Milestones: February 1–February 28 Lose 2 more pounds, for a total of 14 pounds

○ Goal weight on March 1: 136

Comment: I'll be more than halfway there!

Milestones: March 1–March 31 Lose 2 more pounds, for a total of 16 pounds

○ *Goal weight on April 1: 134*

Comment: No fooling: I bet my clothes will be swimming on me

Milestones: April 1–April 30 Lose 2 more pounds, for a total of 18

○ *Goal weight on May 1: 132*

Comment: Take advantage of spring fruits and vegetables for low-cal snacks

Milestones: May 1–May 31 Lose last 2 pounds, for a total of 20

○ *Goal weight on June 1: 130*

Comment: Check out the bathing suit sales

Reviewing Jane's plan

Jane was not reaching too far in her long-term goal. In all likelihood, she will be able to lose a pound a week during the first 8 weeks of her diet. She may lose more than a pound the first week or so and then begin to slow down toward the end, but a total of 8 pounds in 8 weeks is certainly within the realm of the possible.

She was being realistic about the holidays. Anticipating the problems inherent in December, she simply designated it as a plateau. She will be successful if she does not gain any weight during that month.

Knowing the power of a New Year's resolution, she plans to use it to rev up her weight loss. How she will do this remains to be planned.

As winter wanes and spring beckons, she will begin to see a big difference in her shape. By June, she will have reached her goal. She plans to reward herself with a new bathing suit to show off her newly svelte self.

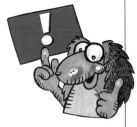

Review your own weight-loss timetable. Look at it carefully and ask yourself: Is it reasonable? Is it feasible?

Measurements optional

As you begin to lose weight, your dimensions will change. Exactly where you lose inches depends on many factors, most of which you have control over. Remember: Spot reducing is a fantasy. Your increased exercise will be firming you up, but you may also gain some inches if you are adding muscular bulk.

Nonetheless, there's nothing more motivating than being able to measure the difference your diet and exercise plan is making. Part of the story will be told by your scale, but you may also want to track changes in your measurements.

If so, take out a tape measure and take off your clothes. Add your starting measurements to your personal database. Here are some you may want to take, but feel free to add others if they are particularly relevant to you.

Losing weight and keeping it off may be harder for me

MY MEASUREMENTS:

Chest/bust	38 in			
Upper thigh	21 in			
Calf	14 in			
Upper arm	14 in			
Lower arm	10 in			
Other				

■ **Write your starting measurements** _in your personal database. After that, measure yourself no more than once a month. It's simply not realistic to expect a noticeable change more often than that._

Your fitness goals

NO MATTER HOW little or how much physical activity you have in your day, it is clearly not enough to fuel your weight loss. If it were, you would not be reading this book. Rather than prescribe a specific amount or type of activity at this point, it is simpler to say: Do more!

Weight loss begins fast and slows down over time. Increasing your activity level should follow the opposite pattern.

Do it little by little

There is nothing worse than going from zero to 90 mph when it comes to exercise. You'll ache all over and be unable to keep it up after the first few days. Gradually add more activity to your day. That will give you a chance to get used to being more active while avoiding injury, charley horses, and generally overdoing it.

WHAT JANE DID

Jane decided to walk to work during the fall days when she began her diet. The half-hour walk was pleasant and not physically taxing. On rainy days, she substituted walking the four flights to her office rather than taking the elevator.

Once the weather got colder, she woke up a half hour earlier and popped an exercise tape into her VCR. She did stretches and calisthenics on Mondays, Wednesdays, and Fridays, and aerobics on Tuesdays, Thursdays, and Saturdays. She took Sunday off.

By February, she had lost enough weight and gained enough confidence to join a gym. She went three times a week, alternating exercise classes with work on the weight machines, but always began with a 15-minute warm-up on the treadmill. Weather permitting, she resumed her walk to work. In bad weather, she took the stairs both at work and at home.

She was pleasantly surprised to find that stair climbing was considerably easier than it had been when she began. She also found she missed the gym on her days off and found herself adding another workout whenever her schedule allowed.

Your plan

YOUR CIRCUMSTANCES *may be similar to Jane's or very different. Jane was very disciplined, and you may not be so. Waking up a half hour earlier each morning may not be possible for you, but eking out a half hour elsewhere in the day may be. Don't let yourself get discouraged if you can't do what Jane did. (After all, I made her up.) Instead, think about how you can gradually add more activity to your day. Start with 15 minutes of something – it really doesn't matter what.*

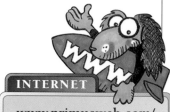

INTERNET

**www.primusweb.com/
fitnesspartner**

If you're short on ideas for increasing activity, take a look at the Fitness Partner Connection. It lists dozens of activities ranging from gym and sports to daily life and occupational activities, along with the calorie burn you'll get according to your weight and the amount of time you do them.

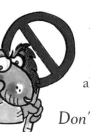

Write down an activity timetable in your notebook. Be sure to indicate the activity you plan to do and the amount of time you plan for each. Provide some alternatives if your activities are weather dependent.

Don't choose activities that are unrealistic for you.

If it takes too much time or is too sweaty for the time of day, you won't do it. If it takes you out of the way or in other ways interferes with your routine, it won't last. If it exhausts you or makes you sore, it's too much. If it's boring, you'll find excuses to avoid it.

Try to add 5 minutes every few days until you are doing a minimum of 30 minutes of something active every day.

By the time you reach this level, you will probably have also reached a weight-loss plateau. And that's when your exercise dividends start to pay off. The activity will be revving up your metabolism, giving your body the extra rpms it needs to keep on burning.

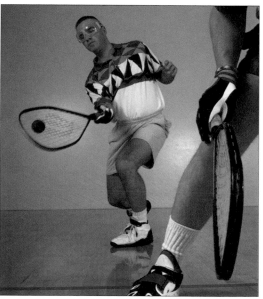

■ **If being outside in the rain or cold** *is your idea of a nightmare, choose a sport that you can play indoors whatever the weather.*

IS NOW THE TIME TO QUIT SMOKING?

This is the crunch point for smokers. You know you need to lose weight. You know you need to quit smoking. Which should you do first? Will doing one make the other problem worse? Wouldn't it just be easier to keep killing yourself?

You have to be the final judge of that, though talking to a doctor or other expert would be a good idea. But here's a radical suggestion: Do both. Now.

If you are really committed to change, really determined to improve your health and appearance, why not take the plunge? The same resolve, the same self-discipline, the same positive energy are required for both. And in a very real sense, the same strategies will work:

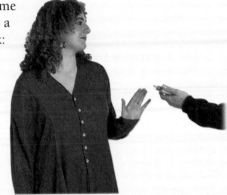

1 Learn as much as you can about the health risks of smoking.

2 Think about it in stages, giving yourself milestones, motivators, and rewards.

3 Make a plan.

4 Put it into action.

■ **Quitting smoking** *is one of the best things you can do for your health* .

Calculating the calories

For every pound you want to lose, you will have to eliminate 3,500 calories. You can do this by eating less, exercising more, or a combination of the two. You know enough by now to guess that the combination is the way to go.

Regardless of your timetable, the 3,500-calorie figure holds. Ten pounds means 35,000 fewer calories, 20 pounds means 70,000 fewer. Stretched out over 6 months (180 days), 200 and 400 fewer calories a day will do it.

Take a look at your food and activity diary pages. Can you knock 100 calories worth of food out of each day and add 100 calories worth of exercise?

Of course you can!

Making a contract

AS CORNY AS IT MAY SEEM, *I strongly urge you to write a weight-loss contract. You can word it anyway you wish, but take a look at Jane's contract for some ideas.*

JANE'S CONTRACT

I, Jane Doe, who currently weighs 150 pounds and has a BMI of 26, hereby resolve to lose 20 pounds and achieve a BMI of 22.

I will do it over the course of 9 months, beginning September 1 and ending June 1 the following year.

I will do it with a combination of calorie reduction and increased activity. My goal is to eliminate 260 calories a day through a combination of these means.

I will lose weight and increase activity according to the attached timetable.

I will review my progress on a weekly basis and reassess my methods on a monthly basis. If I am not achieving my milestones, I will either revise them to be more realistic or further reduce my caloric intake and/or increase my level of activity.

If I achieve my goal before June 1, I will reward myself with a weekend at the beach. If I do not achieve my goal by June 1, I will allow myself a 30-day grace period.

After achieving my goal, I will continue to exercise and eat wisely to ensure that I maintain my weight loss. If I gain more than 2 pounds, I will immediately analyze the causes and reinstate my weight-loss routine.

Signed: Jane Doe   Date:

Witness: Jack Sprat   Date:

Note that Jane has included a schedule for evaluation and reassessment. It may turn out that her goals and timetable were not realistic. Rather than giving up entirely, she has built in the possibility of revision.

She has also given herself an incentive for doing better than she predicted and a grace period if she falls short. Finally, she has written in a pledge to keep off the weight she loses. Jane knows that eating wisely and staying active are lifelong habits, not short-term stratagems.

Take out your notebook and write your own contract. Sign and date it. Get a witness, if you think that will help. Take it with you on your climb and refer to it often.

A simple summary

✔ Self-knowledge is the necessary first step in designing an effective weight-loss plan.

✔ Keeping a food and activity diary is an important way to gain knowledge about your current habits and to see how you can change.

✔ Setting both short- and long-term goals will keep you motivated and realistic.

✔ Your plan should include both reducing caloric intake and increasing caloric use through activity.

✔ Aim to lose a reasonable amount of weight over an extended period of time.

✔ Analyze your plan to be sure it is realistic and feasible, and then review it once a month, making revisions if necessary.

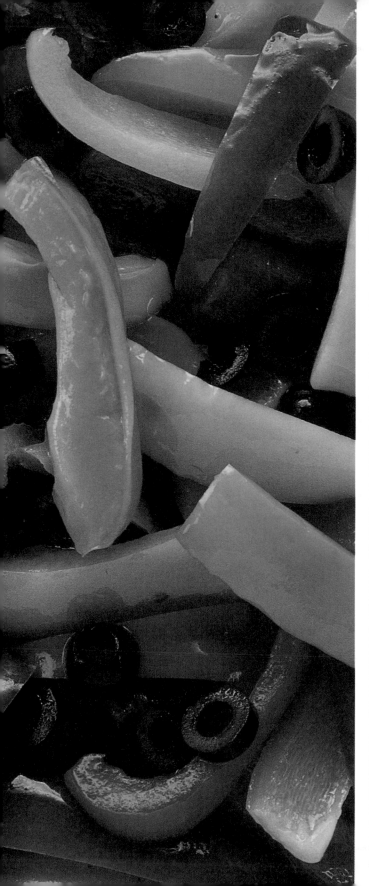

PART FOUR

CRISP VEGETABLES ADD BITE TO A LOW-CAL SALAD

PLANNING IT

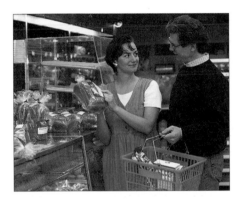

THIS BOOK DOES NOT ESPOUSE a particular diet or weight-loss plan. Instead it assumes that you are an intelligent individual. You know how to take *information* and apply it to your own circumstances, tailor it to your own personality, and focus it on your own problems.

In this section, you'll get information to help you evaluate the range of possibilities offered in books, magazines, commercial programs, and on the World Wide Web. There are warnings about useless, dangerous, and otherwise unhelpful weight-loss schemes, countered with healthy *diet principles*. Find out how to add more activity to your life and get ideas, and support for both eating and exercising for weight-loss. Finally, your own *weight-loss plan* will start you off on the first week of a lifelong program of fitness and health.

Chapter 10

Diet Don'ts

THERE IS NO SIMPLE WAY to lose weight, and certainly not a single diet that will work for everyone. The best, and ultimately the simplest, way to lose weight and keep it off is to understand what works, what doesn't, and why, and then put that knowledge into practice. To put it simply, you need to educate yourself. Sadly, there are a lot of dangerous diets out there, and many others that simply don't work. This chapter is a consumer's guide to fad diets and other weight-loss schemes.

In this chapter...

✓ What's wrong with this diet?

✓ Duck these diet dangers

✓ Special-occasion dieting

✓ Use with care

✓ It's a matter of calories

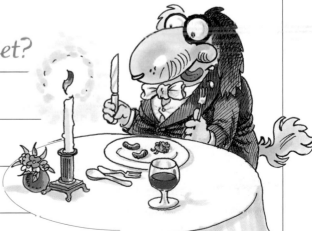

What's wrong with this diet?

IF YOU SPEND ANY TIME *perusing the diet shelves of bookstores, or watching daytime television, or surfing the Internet, you are undoubtedly aware of an avalanche of diets: celebrity diets, low-carbohydrate diets, 3-day diets, diets designed to fit your blood type, astrological sign, age, gender, what have you. Most promise some sort of miracle, something quick and easy. And you may be tempted to give them a try.*

Yo-yo dieting

Most likely, you have dieted before. Maybe you lost a few pounds, maybe you lost many. But the reason you bought this book is that you gained them back again. This is the familiar diet yo-yo.

Although some people say that yo-yo dieting messes up your metabolism and does lasting harm to your health, this is actually not true.

Medical experts call it weight cycling, and this is what they have to say about it:

1. Weight cycling does not have a permanent effect on your metabolic rate.

2. Weight cycling does not increase the amount of your fat tissue.

3. Weight cycling will not turn you into an "apple," causing you to regain lost weight as fat deposits in your abdominal area.

The main thing wrong with yo-yo dieting is that it is discouraging.

And the main cause of yo-yoing is diets that result in temporary weight loss rather than encouraging permanent changes in your eating and exercise habits.

High-protein, high-fat diets

The most popular diets today are based on the premise that being overweight is caused primarily by carbohydrates. These diets call for eating a lot of protein and little or no carbohydrates. Most of them also permit you to eat as much fat as you want. Their promoters claim this is a healthier way of eating.

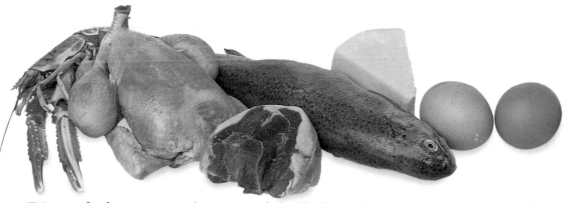

■ **Protein foods** *are an essential component of a healthy, balanced diet. But high-protein, high-fat diets deprive you of vitamins, minerals, fiber, and many more benefits that come with the other food groups.*

You undoubtedly know some people who have lost a great deal of weight, and quite quickly, on these diets. And it is hard to argue with success. But I'm going to do it anyway. High protein, low-carbohydrate diets are extremely unhealthy. The reasons for this are:

1. They violate every known fact about nutritionally balanced eating.

2. They ignore the established health risks of diets high in cholesterol and saturated fats.

3. They overload you with protein, which results in loss of calcium from your bones, which may lead to osteoporosis. Protein overload also puts stress on your kidneys as they try to eliminate large amounts of urea, a by-product of protein metabolism.

4. They forbid foods known to lower the risk of heart disease and many cancers.

5. They deprive you of carbohydrates, the nutrient group most readily converted to energy. Even moderately active people will notice this lack during exercise.

6. They deprive your brain of glucose, which it needs for normal functioning. The result is a slowdown in thinking and reaction time.

7. They deprive you of the enormous benefits of fiber, which is found in carbohydrate-rich foods.

8. They are deficient in essential vitamins.

9. They cause potentially dangerous changes in your body chemistry.

10. They deliver temporary weight loss. Weight gain is rapid once you go off the diet.

Some "carbs are the enemy" diets are based on pseudo-scientific theories about insulin. Carbohydrates do not overstimulate insulin production in people whose insulin-secreting cells function normally. The best way to ensure that you do not have an "insulin problem" is to have a blood glucose test as part of an annual preventive health examination. If your blood sugar level is abnormal, your doctor will investigate the cause and discuss dietary changes with you. If your blood sugar is normal, the healthiest thing you can do is to ensure that 55 to 60 percent of your daily calories come from carbohydrates, primarily complex carbohydrates.

■ **Carbohydrates** *are the nutrients that are most readily converted into energy in the body. Cutting them out of your diet can make you feel tired and lethargic.*

The rapid weight loss seen in people on low-carb diets is mostly due to water loss.

Protein metabolism produces urea, a toxin eliminated in urine through the kidneys. Every gram of urea requires 50 ml of water to flush it from the body. That's a little more than an ounce of water, and remember: A fluid ounce of water weighs an ounce. In addition, fat metabolism produces ketone bodies, another toxin that increases water loss.

INTERNET

www.phys.com

Click on Weight Loss and then "The Diet Debunker," a valuable feature that shines the bright light of reality on all the current fad diets. As a bonus, you'll find tips on "What to tell friends who claim it works" for every diet reviewed.

Very low-calorie diets

One of the main attractions of the high-protein/low-carbohydrate diets is that you can eat all you want, calories be damned. On the other end of the spectrum are very low-calorie diets and, at the most extreme, fasting.

Very low-calorie diets typically restrict you to 1,000 calories a day or less. Aside from the fact that such diets are agony to stay on for more than a few days, they are less effective than you would imagine. The trouble is that your body very soon gets the idea that it's famine time and drops into low gear. Remember back in Chapter 5 when we were talking about metabolic changes? The body's natural response to reduced calories is to adjust metabolism to reduced need.

■ **Eating nothing but celery** *for lunch may seem virtuous, but it won't get you through the day.*

The result is that the lower your caloric intake, the lower your energy. People on very low-calorie diets feel light-headed and weak. Just about all they can manage is to lie around thinking about their next meager meal. Too bad they don't realize that they could be losing more weight, and feeling a lot better, if they ate more and got some exercise.

Do not, under any circumstances, undertake a fast or a very low-calorie diet without medical supervision.

Very low-calorie diets may be appropriate for a short time for severely obese people, who are usually monitored in a hospital setting. For anyone else, they can be dangerous.

■ **Severely limiting calorie intake** *will make you feel weak and listless. It's far more effective to lose weight by eating and exercising more.*

DIETS OF THE RICH AND FAMOUS

We are invited to diet with the Duchess, to do it the Suzanne Sommers way, to adopt the Beverly Hills habit. The main thing these diets have going for them is the fame attached to the name. Unless a diet encourages a long-term change in eating habits and metabolism-boosting exercise, their effect will be as fleeting as, well, fame.

Most of the glamorous folks who put their names on these diets also have access to personal trainers and cosmetic surgeons. I have nothing against personal trainers, if you can afford one, because they'll drive you to exercise hard. As for cosmetic surgery, liposuction is an expensive way to change your looks, not your life.

If a particular celebrity diet is also a sound one, and if you are motivated by emulating a famous person, there is no harm in trying it. But carefully examine the diet behind the name. Like any sensible diet, it should be based on the principle of calories in/calories out. That's the only way to lose weight.

Crash diets

There are 3-day diets, 5-day diets, diets that promise you'll drop a pound a day for 2 weeks. These are very appealing for people who want to lose weight for a special occasion. And they are the leading cause of yo-yo dieting.

Remember: If it's fast, it won't last.

As soon as you go back to eating the way you always have, the pounds will come back. And chances are, they'll come back with a vengeance since the deprivation of the quick diet will have slowed your metabolism, requiring fewer calories and causing your body to store the excess as fat.

These diets claim to "jump start" your weight loss, but in fact they do just the opposite. Going on a quickie diet implies going off it. You haven't changed your eating habits. You haven't incorporated more activity into your day. All you've done is temporarily forced your metabolism into starvation mode.

Other nutritionally unbalanced diets

Diets that prescribe a single category of food are just plain unhealthy. It doesn't matter if it's only grains or only greens or only meat. You need some of all of the major nutrient groups, in the proportions outlined in Chapter 4. To review:

1. A balanced diet for an adult should derive 55 to 60 percent of its calories from carbohydrates, most of them complex carbohydrates.

2. The average adult needs about half a gram of protein for every pound of body weight.

3. Even fat is essential, but it should make up no more than 30 percent of your daily caloric intake, and most of it should be unsaturated.

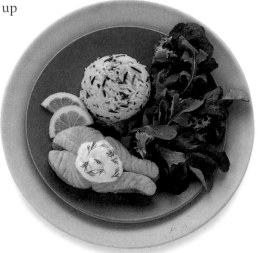

■ **A nutritionally balanced** *diet will provide all the vitamins and minerals you need. Nutritionally unbalanced diets risk not only malnutrition, but also vitamin and mineral deficiencies that can lead to serious health problems.*

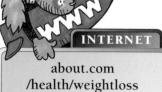

INTERNET

about.com /health/weightloss

Click on Doubtful Diets if you're still in doubt.

Duck these diet dangers

"QUACK, QUACK!" That's the sound of weight-loss fraud. It comes out of health food stores and the Internet. It blasts from the front pages of supermarket tabloids. If you're like me, your e-mailbox is filled with it. Everywhere you turn today, someone is trying to sell you an easy weight-loss dream.

False promises

There is no such thing as the "Mayo Clinic Diet." Several diets go by that name, but they're all imposters. Some claim that eating grapefruit before each meal will act as a "fat catalyst." Another promises a weight loss of more than 50 pounds in 2 months. Others are heavy on saturated fats and cholesterol. Whatever the diet, it's totally bogus. It has nothing to do with the respected Mayo Clinic. It will not help you lose weight. It is not healthy.

INTERNET

www.mayo.edu/ about.mayo_diet.html

If you want to know what the Mayo Clinic has to say about the so-called Mayo Clinic Diet, log on to this page. Or click on the link to "Ask the Mayo Dietician," which contains not only an answer to the "Mayo Diet" claims, but also lots of good advice on healthy eating and weight loss.

My mother sent me a brochure she received for "miracle fat-melting" asparagus pills. Personally, I prefer my asparagus steamed whole. I used to like them cloaked in hollandaise, but now I find the taste is better with a squeeze of lemon.

You may be amused (or appalled) to read this slice of spam I recently received. I reproduce the best parts here (complete with grammatical errors and creative capitalization).

"Have you heard enough about ALL of them low, or restricted carbohydrate diets and are interested in trying it out for yourself? Would you like to try out this latest new "diet" rage but don't have time to read the books? If so, this e-mail was MEANT FOR YOU!

"I have put together my OWN MENU . . . Using this one of a kind 14 DAY MENU, I LOST 23 POUNDS in just SIX weeks, and have kept it off AND have maintained my ideal body COMPOSITION since Aug, 1999! Not only did eating less carbohydrates make my body use up my stored fats, my energy level SOARED after only 2 weeks! One of the best things is that my cholesterol actually DROPPED while not giving up MEAT!

"For ONLY $10 USD, I will send you my very own, 14 DAY "restricted carbo" MENU!

"Being a lover of FOOD (everything!), you will NEVER go hungry on my plan!
"Of course, exercise is always encouraged, however it wasn't part of my daily activity...
"Losing them unwanted pounds and flab WILL change your life, just like it has for me!"

Words of wisdom

Okay, spotting the hoax behind the hype was easy on this one, but how can you tell about the many others? Here's what the Food and Drug Administration and Federal Trade Commission advise.

Be skeptical about any weight-loss scheme that claims to be:

- easy
- effortless
- guaranteed
- magical
- miraculous
- exclusive
- a new discovery
- mysterious
- exotic
- secret
- a breakthrough
- ancient

Beware of such weight-loss "wonders" as:

- diet patches
- starch blockers
- glucomannan and other bulk producers
- appetite-suppressing eyeglasses
- electrical muscle stimulators for weight loss
- fat blockers
- magnet pills
- spirulina
- magic weight-loss earrings

Appetite-suppressing eyeglasses and magic weight-loss earrings??? Gimme a break!

Laxatives, enemas, and *emetics* are easy to come by over the counter, and they are a favorite "diet aid" of people with eating disorders. Used frequently, they can do serious damage to the intestines, esophagus, and tooth enamel. Mineral oil is another popular but dangerous strategy. By interfering with absorption of fat-soluble vitamins, its use can result in serious vitamin deficiency.

Laxatives, enemas, emetics, and mineral oil have no place in a weight-loss program — they can be dangerous to health.

If you do use any "diet aids", discuss the health implications with your doctor without delay.

DEFINITION

An emetic is something that induces vomiting. Ipecac is one emetic that is available without a prescription. Pressing down on the back of the tongue may also induce vomiting. In addition to food, vomiting brings up stomach acid, which can burn the delicate tissues of the throat and mouth and erode tooth enamel.

DIET SUPPLEMENTS

I have already spoken about the dangers of some over-the-counter products sold as dietary supplements. Not all are intended to help you lose weight, but many are. What they all have in common is their ability to slip through a regulatory loophole that permits them to be sold without a prescription as long as they do not claim to cure any disease or condition. Their makers do not have to prove that they are either safe or effective, as the manufacturers of licensed drugs have to. There is no safeguard against the inclusion of dangerous ingredients or contamination during the manufacturing process. Nor is there any guarantee that the ingredients on the label are present in the amounts indicated – if at all. The dangers of overdosing and creating chemical and nutritional imbalances are real.

Some supplements claim to melt away fat or prevent its absorption from food. Others promise to boost your metabolism. Yet others say they will increase your energy. Body builders are encouraged to supplement their exercise routine with pills and powders to increase their strength and muscle mass.

Here's a "most unwanted" list of diet supplement ingredients you should stay away from.

Muscle builders:
- androstenedione
- beta-hydroxy-beta-methylbutrate (HMB)
- dehydroepiandrosterone (DHEA)
- pyruvate
- inosine
- choline
- glandular extracts
- vitamin B12 as dibencobal and cyanocobalamin
- magnesium

Amino acids:
- creatine
- ornithine
- lysine
- arginine
- inosine
- leucine
- tyrosine
- glutamine

Fat burners:
- carnitine
- chromium

If you take these supplements, you are wasting time and money, and risking your health.

Special-occasion dieting

SUMMER IS COMING and the thought of you in a bathing suit spells a-w-f-u-l. New Year's Eve and a little black dress beckons. Your high school reunion is a month away and you've gained a pound for every year since you graduated. Wouldn't it be nice to lose 10 pounds for such occasions?

It would be nice, and it would even be feasible if you do it right.

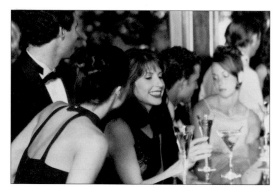

■ **If a party or special occasion** *motivates you to lose weight, that's great, but remember that you have to remain motivated to keep the weight off.*

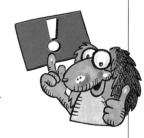

Dieting for a special occasion works only if it's part of an overall plan to change the way you eat and exercise over the long term.

If dieting for a special occasion motivates you to get started, great. If you drop your plan as soon as you drop 10 pounds, not so great. The same principles apply to special-occasion dieting as to a lifelong plan.

1. You need to be realistic about how much you want to lose and how long you will take to do it.

2. You need to take a good look at what's keeping you over your desired weight and resolve to change those habits and behaviors.

3. You need to design a healthy eating plan that you will be able to live with over the long term.

4. You need to incorporate more physical activity in your day, to burn calories and keep your metabolism humming as your energy needs drop along with your weight.

Do not think of a diet as a quick fix for a temporary problem.

You may be able to squeeze into that dress on New Year's Eve, but if you don't also make and keep some resolutions, you'll have to do it all over again for the reunion and again to make the most of the summer sun.

Use with care

IF YOUR WEIGHT-LOSS STRATEGY *includes reducing the number of calories you consume, you may be attracted to low-cal substitutes for sugar and fat. There's a good reason why diet soft drinks are perennial bestsellers, but they are not necessarily the dieter's best friend.*

Sugar substitutes

Saccharin and aspartame are the two most common sugar replacements. You can buy them separately or find them in a vast array of low-cal, no-cal, and diet products, from gum and candy to soda, ice cream, and more.

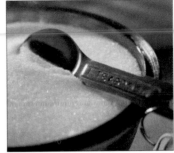

Both saccharin and aspartame have long been the subjects of controversy over their safety. I won't get into the complex and heated arguments about this, since it could fill a book. To keep it simple, they should be used, if at all, in moderation. Health issues aside, using artificial sweeteners is not a way to deal with a sweet tooth. If you crave sweet foods, it would be better to try to understand why. Are you using them to fill an emotional need? Is reaching for a sweet a habit you can break or at least modify?

■ **Sugar substitutes** *may taste like the real thing, but they're not the cure for a sweet tooth.*

If you like sugary drinks and other sweet foods, compare the calorie content of what you eat when your food is sweetened with sugar and when it is sweetened artificially.

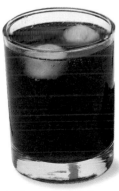

How much of your daily calorie intake are you "saving" by using a sugar substitute? Can you think of other ways to save these calories? Use your food diary to make this analysis, then consider modifying your dependence on these additives by reducing sweets in general and alternating sugar and its substitutes when you do want, or need, a sweet.

Artificial sweeteners, however, are a boon for people with diabetes, who must watch their sugar consumption carefully.

■ **Diet soft drinks** *are big sellers, but they're best enjoyed in moderation.*

If you have diabetes, discuss your consumption of artificial sweeteners with your doctor.

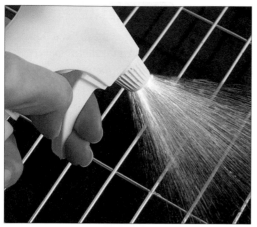

■ **Using non-stick coatings** *or oil-water sprays keeps food from sticking to a grill or frying pan without adding calories.*

Fat substitutes

Depending on what you want from dietary fat, there are a number of substitutes designed to help. Low- or no-cal butter flavoring is an option if what you want is the taste. Not everyone can't believe it's not butter, however. Nonstick coatings and sprays don't add flavor or the distinctive "mouth feel" of fat. And therein lies the rub.

Much of the flavor and succulence of food comes courtesy of fat.

Finding other ways to make food flavorful and texturally appealing is the obvious solution, and we will be talking about how to do that in Chapter 15. But thanks to the miracle of modern science, some fat substitutes have been developed so you can have your fat and eat it too.

One of these is called olestra, a synthetic fat with zero calories. It behaves like natural oils and fats when used for cooking. It was approved by the FDA for use in such snack foods as chips and crackers, which are available on your supermarket shelf.

Unfortunately, the very thing that makes olestra a no-calorie wonder makes it somewhat problematic. Similar to the prescription fat-blocker orlistat, olestra causes some unpleasant changes in the behavior of your bowels, including abdominal cramps, flatulence, diarrhea, urgent and oily stools, and what has been delicately described as anal leakage. It also interferes with the absorption of fat-soluble vitamins (A, D, E, K) and beta-carotene.

Orlistat is taken in prescribed doses, but if you are a dedicated snacker, you could down a huge bag of olestra-laced potato chips in one sitting. You might think you were getting away like a low-cal, low-fat bandit, but your digestive system will tell you otherwise.

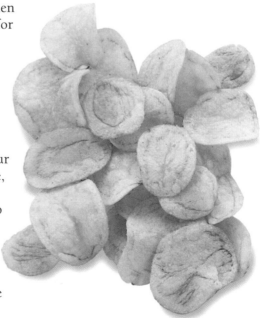

■ **Potato chips** *that won't make you fat sound a great idea, but your digestive system may disagree.*

Cholesterol-lowering foods

The second new development is not technically a fat substitute. It combines unsaturated vegetable oils with a substance derived from plants that has been found to lower cholesterol. You'll find this substance in Take Control margarine and a line of foods under the label Benecol, which includes both margarine and a variety of snack foods. Unlike olestra, these "designer fats" do contain calories your body can absorb. (Check the package label for the exact per serving calorie count of anything you're considering trying.) The major attraction is their effect on "bad cholesterol."

The cholesterol-lowering effect lasts only as long as you "take" these foods. In fact, they are so much like medicine that some experts think they should be classified that way. The FDA has recently made that argument and it remains to be seen how and whether these *functional foods* will be regulated in the future.

As with sugar substitutes, fat substitutes do not help you change your eating habits.

Using them to replace some of the fat in your diet is not the same as developing a taste for less fatty foods. My advice on these substitutes is to use them with care if you must use them at all. If you have high cholesterol, talk to your doctor about the role "cholesterol-lowering" foods should have in your overall health strategy.

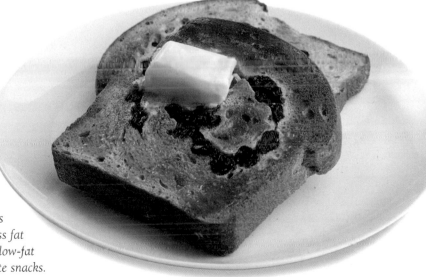

■ **Fat substitutes,** *such as margarine, contain the same number of calories as butter. The key is to use less fat altogether, and to think of low-fat alternatives to your favorite snacks.*

It's a matter of calories

ANALYZE ANY DIET *that succeeds in making you lose weight and you will find that it supplies you with fewer calories than your body needs. Highly prescriptive diets – that is, those that tell you exactly what and how much you can eat – work their "magic" by restricting calories. It's not the cabbage or the grapefruit or your blood type or the zone you're in. It's not the specific combination of foods or the order in which you eat them.*

It is, plain and simple, a matter of calories. All together now:

1 If you consume more calories than you use, you will gain weight.

2 If you use more calories than you consume, you will lose weight.

No matter what alchemy is claimed by the hawkers of miracle fad diets, and even low-cal substitutes, it all comes down to calories.

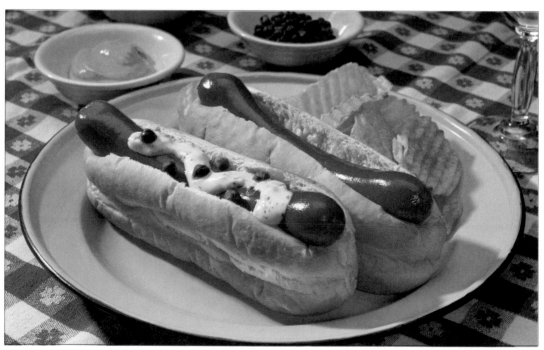

■ **Two hotdogs, potato chips, mayonnaise, and counting.** *That's a lot of calories in total, and if you're not expending them, you'll be storing them as fat.*

A simple summary

✔ Losing and regaining weight in cycles is discouraging, but it will not alter your metabolism or otherwise damage your health.

✔ Quick weight loss on fad diets is invariably followed by quick weight gain as soon as the diet is over.

✔ High protein, high-fat diets that forbid or drastically limit carbohydrates are unhealthy and dangerous.

✔ Fasting and very low-calorie diets should be undertaken only by severely obese people under medical supervision.

✔ Nutritionally unbalanced diets are difficult, and dangerous, to keep up over the long-term.

✔ Weight loss is always, and only, the result of caloric intake that is less than caloric output.

✔ Miracle weight-loss schemes waste your money and time, and may even risk your health. Don't be fooled by hype, no matter how persuasive.

✔ Weight loss supplements without a prescription are not studied or tested for safety and effectiveness.

✔ Dieting for a special occasion makes sense only if it motivates you to change your eating and exercise habits over the long term.

✔ Sugar and fat substitutes will not help you to change your eating habits and are no substitute for sensible eating. Use them sparingly, if at all.

✔ There is no secret – ancient or cutting edge – to weight loss. "Calories-in, calories-out" is the rule.

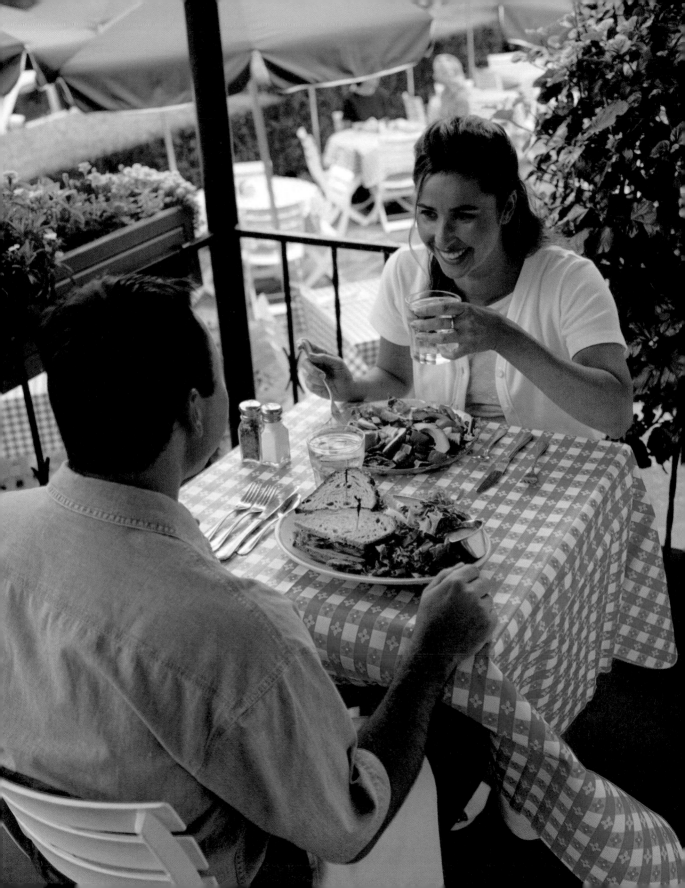

Chapter 11

Diet Right

Now that you know what doesn't work when it comes to weight loss, you're probably wondering what does. Quite simply, any diet you choose should be based on scientifically valid and healthy principles. In this chapter, I will lay out healthy diet principles and give you some real-life examples of how to put them into practice. Because the focus is on you – your eating habits, your goals, your weight loss – we'll end the chapter by revising your food diary based on what you've learned.

In this chapter...

✓ Healthy diet principles

✓ Pick complex carbohydrates

✓ Diet smart strategies

✓ A scavenger hunt

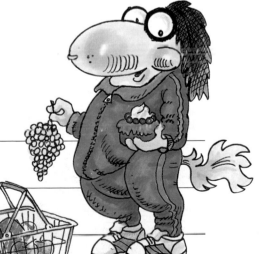

DIETING IS NOT ABOUT DEPRIVATION, IT'S ABOUT EATING AND ENJOYING THE RIGHT FOODS

Healthy diet principles

WEIGHT LOSS SHOULD BE GRADUAL. It should result from realistic changes in the way you eat rather than short but intense bursts of deprivation. A diet that works is a diet you can live with over the long term. That's the only way to ensure that the weight you worked so hard to lose stays lost.

If you don't already have one, go out and buy a calorie counter.

You'll find a wide selection in bookstores. Many supermarkets carry them on the racks near the cash register. Even though calorie counters are available on the Internet, having something you can carry around with you will be invaluable. Before you buy, look up a few of your favorite foods and see if they are listed. Try to find a counter that tells you the fat, protein, and carbohydrate content of each food in addition to the calorie count. Most calorie counters include many foods by brand. If you eat a lot of fast food, there are even calorie counters that specialize in that.

It goes without saying, however, that you should re-examine your habit of eating fast foods, which tend to be loaded with fat, salt, and other unhealthful ingredients.

For those serious about losing weight, fast foods are out.

Calories do count

The only way to lose weight is to take in fewer calories than your body needs for basic functions and daily activities. You know that already, right? You can do it by reducing the number of calories you eat. It's easiest to do this on a daily basis, but overeating one day can be corrected by eating less on subsequent days. You can do it by increasing your level of physical activity so you burn more calories. A small increase every day is easier, and safer, than an all-out effort once or twice a week.

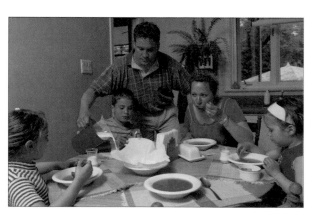

■ **Enlist your family's** *support in your weight-loss campaign – more healthful eating habits will benefit them, too.*

The best way to lose weight is to combine reduced calorie intake with increased activity. And the best way to ensure that this becomes a lifelong habit is to make eating and exercise choices that fit your temperament, preferences, and schedule.

Cut the fat

Fat contains more than double the calories of carbohydrate and protein. You simply get more for your (calorie) money when you tip the balance away from fats. Doing so is also much better for your health. Many fatty foods contain saturated fats, which increase levels of bad cholesterol. That puts you at risk for serious health problems. There are a lot of ways to reduce the fat in what you eat. You'll probably want to try them all.

Go the low-fat route

There are lower-fat equivalents for many foods. Substituting these for high-fat foods is an easy way to reduce the fat. For example, milk, yogurt, cottage cheese, cream cheese, and many other cheeses come in fat percentages ranging from four percent to zero percent. The calorie difference can be significant. Take milk, for example.

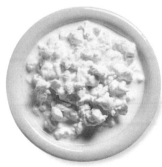

% fat	calories per 8 oz. serving
4 (whole)	150
2 (reduced fat)	130
1 (low-fat)	110
0 (non-fat or skim)	90

■ **Low-fat cottage cheese** *makes a tasty topping for crackers, and is far lower in calories than higher-fat cheeses.*

Find a substitute

Another way to reduce fat is to substitute one food for another. For example, sour cream has 30 calories per tablespoon, whereas the same amount of plain low-fat yogurt has only 9 calories. A tablespoon of mayonnaise, made from oil and eggs, has 100 calories, whereas ketchup has 16 and mustard has 5. Lemon juice has 4 calories per tablespoon and soy sauce has 10. Keep these values in mind when you are thinking about dressings and toppings to add interest and flavor to food. Fish and meat come in a wide range from fatty to lean. Educate yourself about the per-serving calorie counts of these protein sources.

When it comes to fish, in general, the lighter the meat's color, the lower the fat content.

Cod, flounder, and other white fish have 1 gram of fat per 4-ounce serving. The same amount of pale fish like catfish, pink salmon, and swordfish has 5 grams of fat. Dark fish like bluefish, red salmon, and mackerel have 16 grams of fat.

TAKE IT OFF

Remove all visible fat from food before you eat it. It's best to take off the fat before you cook it. Take the skin off fish, or buy it skinless. It's also a good idea to skim fat from all soups, gravies, and sauces. Fat rises to the top of liquids and is easy to scrape off when soup, gravy, or sauce has been refrigerated until the fat solidifies.

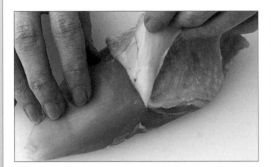

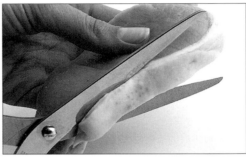

a **Skin chicken breasts**

Get a good grip on one edge of the skin and pull, then use scissors or a knife to trim off all traces of skin and get rid of any globs of fat.

b **Trim the fat from meat**

For chops and similar cuts of meat, use kitchen scissors to remove the fat. Remember that it's better to trim off some meat than leave any fat.

Choose oil-free versions

Dry-roasted nuts and water-packed tuna and other canned fish are obviously the way to go. A six-ounce can of chunk light tuna packed in water has 1.5 grams of fat and 150 calories; packed in oil, the count is 14 grams of fat and 275 calories, and that's *after* the oil has been drained away. After a while, you won't even like the taste of the oily kind.

Cook it right

The cooking method you choose can help reduce fat. Say good-bye to frying and sautéing. Gravies and sauces made from pan drippings are also taboo. You can steam, boil, or poach foods without adding fat. Baking or broiling over a rack allows fat to drip out of food and into a pan below it. Microwaving is a real boon, since the moisture in food does the cooking, requiring no added fat. Foods that can be eaten raw – especially vegetables – are crisp and delicious without added fat.

Buy yourself a steamer and heatproof rack. If you plan to use them in a microwave, get nonmetallic ones.

A VOCABULARY LESSON

Low fat, reduced fat, fat free. What's the difference? Well, there's a big difference, but unless you know the lingo, you may be fooled into thinking you're cutting more fat than you actually are. Here are the FDA definitions:

- **Fat free** means less than half a gram of fat per serving.
- **Low fat** means 3 grams of fat or less per serving.
- **Reduced fat** means 25 percent less fat than the regular product.

When it comes to foods with less fat, caveat emptor (and eater)!

Reduced-fat bologna is not a low-fat or low-calorie food; neither is reduced-fat bacon or cheese. For example, a slice of regular bacon has 13 grams of fat. A reduced-fat slice would have a little less than 10 grams of fat. That's still 90 calories worth of fat alone!

If you read the label, you may find many examples such as these:

- **Fat-free fig cookies** that have 20 calories more per cookie, than the regular kind.
- **Reduced-fat peanut butter** with exactly the same calorie count as regular.
- **Nonfat ice cream** with 10 more calories per serving than regular.

The moral? Read the label.

None of these terms tells you anything about calorie count, but the FDA has rules about that too.

- **Low caloric** means 40 calories or less per serving.
- **Light (or lite)** means one-third fewer calories or 50 percent less fat than the regular product.

The same warning applies to light/lite foods. Light ice cream will never give a bowl of strawberries a run for its money. A typical half cup of regular ice cream has 10 grams of fat and 160 calories; the light version has 4 grams of fat and 140 calories. And the strawberries? A whole cup has 45 calories and no fat. At that rate, you could top it with a tablespoon of whipped cream (1 gram fat, 10 calories) and still come out way ahead.

Pick complex carbohydrates

CARBOHYDRATES HAVE FEWER *than half the calories of fat. They also make you feel fuller. And it goes without saying that they are far healthier than fat.*

A new way of thinking about this relies on something called *calorie density*. It's really just the same old idea that carbohydrates are higher in bulk than fats and proteins. Three ounces of lettuce has 5 to 10 calories; 3 ounces of steak has about 200. Which has a greater calorie density? Good for you: You passed the math test.

Vegetables, fruits, and grains are all excellent sources of complex carbohydrates. They are low- or nonfat foods and can be prepared in many ways that require the addition of little or no fat.

The food pyramid recommends at least five servings of fruits and vegetables a day.

Because these tend to be high-bulk, low-calorie foods, you'll do well to eat even more than that.

Grains and grain products are especially good choices for weight loss. They are low in fat and make you feel full.

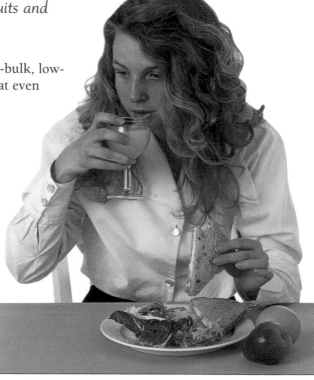

■ **A sandwich** *of wholegrain bread and a low-fat filling, salad, and some fruit is a satisfying meal with a good nutrient balance. Choosing juice over water or another low-calorie beverage may not be the wisest choice however, since fruit is high in sugar.*

Limit sweets

Sugar is a carbohydrate, but not the healthy kind. It is devoid of vitamins, minerals, and fiber. As a source of calories, it's really no bargain. Remember the position sugar and other sweets occupy on the food pyramid. As with fat, you can reduce sugar with a combination of strategies.

1 **Try sugar substitutes:** Within limits, aspartame and saccharin will help you satisfy your sweet tooth without adding calories. They should be used in moderation.

2 **Have just a little:** If you have a craving for sweets, eat only enough to satisfy the craving. Maybe just a morsel or a spoonful will do the trick. Stop after you've had a bit and ask yourself if it's enough.

3 **Try something different:** If you get most of your sweets in snacks and desserts, consider something salty or crunchy or delicious in another way. A few pretzels may be just as satisfying as a donut. A slice of melon might end the meal as nicely as a slice of pie.

If your morning cereal is packed with sugar, try a type with no sugar added and toss in a sliced banana or some raisins. This probably won't reduce your breakfast calories, but you'll be trading "empty" sugar calories for calories that come with fiber, vitamins, and minerals.

Remember that sugar goes under many names besides sucrose. Look back at the list of sugar aliases on page 86, Chapter 4, and use it when you read the label on the sweets you eat.

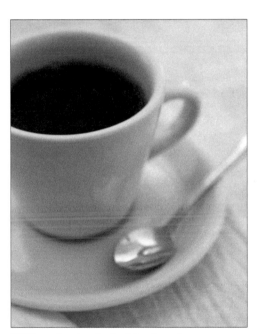

■ **If you're in the habit** *of putting two teaspoons of sugar in your coffee, try it with just one. Chances are, it'll be sweet enough.*

Diet-smart strategies

SHIFTING THE BALANCE *from fats to carbohydrates will have the biggest impact on your calorie intake, but there are many other things you can do to make your diet easier to live with over the long term. Here's a grab bag of good habits that will make you a smarter and more successful weight loser.*

Read the label

Ignorance is no excuse. Thanks to food-labeling laws, there's a wealth of information on every package of prepared food you buy. The three most important items for you to focus on are:

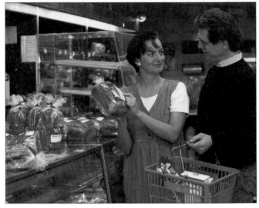

■ **Get into the habit** *of examining food labels at the supermarket: Look at the product's fat content per serving and if it's too high, don't buy!*

1 **Serving size:** There's no point in fooling yourself that you ate only a serving of dessert when you spooned out more than a cup of vanilla fudge ice cream or gobbled a quarter of the cherry pie. Find out what constitutes a serving, and if you eat more than one, face up to that fact.

2 **Calories per serving:** Obviously, oranges and bananas and chicken wings don't come with this information, but packaged food does. This information saves you from having to look up the food in your calorie counter. But it's not worth anything if you ignore serving size.

3 **Grams and percentage of fat:** Each gram of fat is worth 9 calories, as you know. The fat percentage is the best indicator of whether an item is a high-fat food.

Make it satisfying

Think about bulk and texture when you plan your meals. Calorie-dense foods do not satisfy hunger as well as foods that deliver more bulk per calorie. Cheese and crackers can run you 200 calories or more, depending on the type, for only three canapés. A heaping plate of carrots (33 calories for 3 ounces) and sweet peppers (35 calories for 5 ounces) dipped in a quarter cup of salsa (about 30 calories) make a good appetizer, and it adds up to less than half that amount of calories in the cheese and crackers. A 3-ounce slice of chocolate cake will cost you about 350 calories. Mixed fresh fruit salad is a sweet way to end a meal, at only 120 calories per cup.

Fiber is the key here. Grains and fresh fruits and vegetables will make you feel fuller longer than foods that consist primarily of fats, sugar, and protein. Be sure you include fiber-rich foods in every meal you eat.

Texture is another satisfier. Three squares of diet shake a day won't do the trick. When you're planning meals, think about foods that are crunchy, chewy, juicy, smooth, crisp, gooey, succulent, soothing, whatever it is you like.

Simply take your time

Eating slowly is a great weight-loss strategy. It takes about 20 minutes for the "I'm full" signal to get to your brain. If you're chowing down at top speed, the calories will whiz by before the message gets through.

Make it appetizing

If your idea of seasoning is a pat of butter or a dollop of mayo, introduce yourself to the wide world of lower-calorie flavor enhancers. Fresh herbs and spices, flavored vinegars, mustard, lemon juice, soy sauce, marinades, poaching liquids, rubs, and infusions are all ways to add flavor to your food. Being "on a diet" doesn't have to mean deprivation. Let it be an invitation to be more inventive about cooking and food preparation.

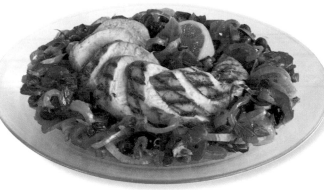

■ **Take a look** at food magazines to see how a small plate with not much food on it can look like a princely feast.

Another way to keep yourself from feeling deprived is to enhance the appearance of the food you eat. Don't just plunk it on your plate. Think about colors and shapes. Arrange things in a pleasing manner.

INTERNET

4weightloss.com

This multipurpose site has a link to several magazines where you'll find lots of weight-wise cooking advice.

Keep it new

There's nothing like the "same old thing" to set your mind wandering where it shouldn't . . . chocolate cake . . . fried fish and chips . . . thick shakes. If what you eat is boring, what you can't eat will be all the more alluring. There is an enormous range of foods you can safely eat. Don't get stuck in a rut. Look in cookbooks and magazines for ideas, and go for variety.

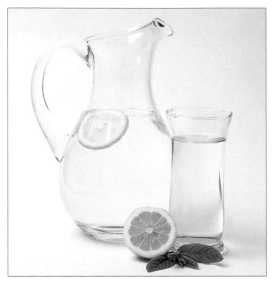

Drink lots of water

Water is your weight-loss ally. You need it to help flush the waste produced by weight loss, but it will also help you feel full. Aim for a minimum of eight glasses a day. Keep track of how much you drink in your food diary. If you have trouble doing this, measure out your daily minimum in bottles. Keep some in the refrigerator, carry one with you whenever you are away from home. When the bottles are empty, you know you've had your fill.

Any time you think you're hungry, drink some water first and then ask yourself whether the hunger is still there.

■ **When you're thirsty**, *reach for no-cal water instead of juice or a soft drink, which can cost you 100 calories a glass, or more.*

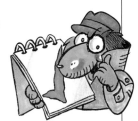

A scavenger hunt

REMEMBER THOSE HUNTS *you used to do with your friends when you were a kid? Well, this one is designed to find the extra calories in your daily food intake. When you're done, you'll have a pretty good idea how you can change the way you eat.*

Take out your weight-loss notebook and your calorie counter. If you bought the kind that lists fat content, your job will be easier. If you did not, check one of the online calorie counters. Many list fat content as well.

Finding the fat

Do you know where the fat is in your diet? You have to find it before you can reduce it. On a separate sheet in your notebook, write the fat content of everything you ate on one of the days in your food diary. To be fair, choose a fairly typical day. If you want to take the time, it will be even more revealing to do it for the entire week.

INTERNET

www.cyberdiet.com

I bet there isn't a food you can't find in the "Database of Foods." You'll get full nutritional info – including calories and grams of fat, but much more – on any quantity of anything you've ever dreamed of eating.

BREAKFAST

		Calories	Fat content
coffee	1 cup	5	0 g
whole milk	1 oz.	20	1 g
plain bagel	med. (3 oz.)	210	2 g
cream cheese	1 oz.	100	10 g
orange juice	8 oz.	110	0 g
Total		475	13 g

Calories from fat:	13g x 9 cal = 117 cal
Fat percentage:	117 ÷ 475 = ·24 (or 24%)

■ **To figure out fat percentage**, *multiply the total grams of fat by 9. (Each gram has 9 calories.) Divide that number by the total calories you consumed. The fat percentage for this breakfast is within desirable limits, but can this person keep it up all day? Is your answer more than 30 percent? If so, you are eating more fat than is healthy for you.*

Keeping fat down

Your aim should be to get the fat percentage of your diet down to 30 percent.

If fat already constitutes 30 percent of your diet, try to get it to 20 percent. Of course, if your total caloric intake is way above your daily needs, 30 percent will add up to a lot of fat. You'll have to cut carbohydrate and protein calories too.

QUICK FAT CALORIE CHECK

Don't want to do the math? Check your fat calories against this chart.

Converting percentage of calories to grams of fat:

Total daily calories	20%	grams fat	30%	grams fat
1,000	200	22	300	33
1,500	300	33	450	50
2,000	400	44	600	65
2,500	500	55	750	80
3,000	600	65	900	100

Look at your food diary again and find as many ways as you can to reduce the fat in what you ate. Lower-fat equivalents or substitutes? A different cooking method? Use your calorie counter and add up the calories for each "revised" meal. How many calories have you knocked off a typical day? A typical week? You'll be surprised at just how much you can cut back with relatively little effort.

Searching for the sweets

Do the same with sweets you ate. How many sugary calories did you pack into a typical day? Don't forget the snacks and soft drinks. And if you pop a mint or hard candy several times a day, be sure to count every last one.

If sweets represent more than 5 percent of your daily calorie intake, your sweet tooth is getting the better of you. How many calories can you eliminate by just saying no? How many can you substitute with artificial sweeteners?

Do not rely on artificially sweetened foods as an answer to reducing your sugar intake. Used in moderation, these are okay, but if you're using diet sodas and candy as a crutch, it's not really healthy.

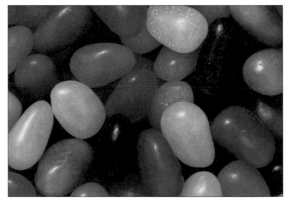

■ **If you're tempted by sweets,** *remember that they reside at the tip of the food pyramid, and so should be eaten sparingly.*

Pinning down the protein

It's important to eat enough protein, but you may be eating more than you need. Look back at the protein RDA table in Chapter 4 (page 76). A simpler way to make sure you're eating enough protein is to look at the food pyramid. As long as you have two to three servings from the meat/poultry/fish/nuts/legumes group each day, you're doing fine. If you eat more than that, you may be overdoing it.

Most Americans eat more than twice the amount of protein they need. Unless you're not eating enough protein, consider cutting down your consumption.

Except for legumes, most protein-rich foods are also sources of fat.

Collecting the carbs

Let's look at that food diary again. Can you replace some of the fatty and sugary foods with a carbohydrate substitute? Can you eat more vegetables or grains and less meat? Would an apple have satisfied your urge to eat as well as those cookies? Would eating a salad before the pizza have allowed you to stop after one slice? Would a mixed-grain pilaf next to one lamb chop have filled your plate and your stomach as much as two lamb chops with a side of pan-roasted potatoes?

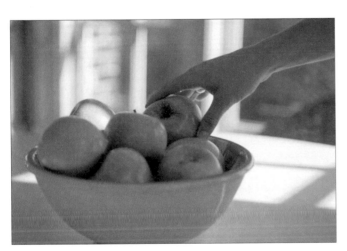

■ **Reach for an apple** *rather than a cookie when you get a hunger pang. It'll satisfy you just as well and it won't pile on the pounds.*

Between 55 and 60 percent of your daily calorie intake should be from carbohydrates, and most of them should be complex carbohydrates (not sugars).

To work out how much of your daily calorie intake is made up of carbohydrates, take out your food diary and do the math on a separate sheet of paper, just as you did when you were finding the fat. For an example of how to do this, turn to the next page.

BREAKFAST

		Calories	Carbohydrates
coffee	1 cup	5	1 g
whole milk	1 oz	20	1.5 g
plain bagel	med. (3 oz)	240	45 g
cream cheese	1 oz	100	1 g
orange juice	8 oz	110	26 g
Total		475	74.5 g

Calories from carbohydrate:	74.5 g x 4 cal = 298
Carbohydrate percentage:	298 ÷ 475 = .627 (nearly 63%)

■ **To figure out carbohydrate percentage,** *multiply the total grams of carbohydrate by 5. (Each gram has 5 calories.) Divide that number by the total calories you consumed. The example scores about 63 percent. Enough carbohydrates, but an awful lot of them are from sugar!*

The bottom line

Add up the total number of calories you think you can eliminate from your food diary day or week by cutting fat and sweets. If you did only a day, multiply by 7. Are you anywhere near 3,500? Are you over that figure? How many days or weeks will it take to subtract 3,500 calories? Each 3,500 unit equals a pound.

Here's the simple truth: If you did absolutely nothing else beyond following the healthy diet principles when you shop, cook, and eat, you'd lose a pound for every 3,500 calories saved.

But there is, in fact, much more you can do. It begins with exercise, which we'll be talking about in the next chapter. And it continues with menu planning and behavior modification, which we'll look at in Chapter 14.

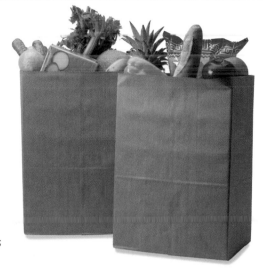

■ **Following healthy diet** *principles when you shop will help you lose weight. You could save a lot of calories simply by avoiding high-fat foods.*

A simple summary

✔ Calories count. Calories count. Calories count.

✔ The only way to lose weight safely is to take in fewer calories than your body uses.

✔ Weight loss should always be gradual. Slow and steady weight loss is your best insurance against rapid weight gain.

✔ Cutting fat, limiting sweets, and choosing complex carbohydrates as your primary foods are the most important healthy diet principles.

✔ Reducing fat is the most effective way to reduce calories.

✔ A diet rich in complex carbohydrates is a satisfying way to reduce calories without going hungry.

✔ Dieting need not mean deprivation. Planning meals that are delicious, attractive, and satisfying will help you develop lifelong healthy eating habits.

✔ Reading food labels and paying attention to serving size are very important calorie-control strategies.

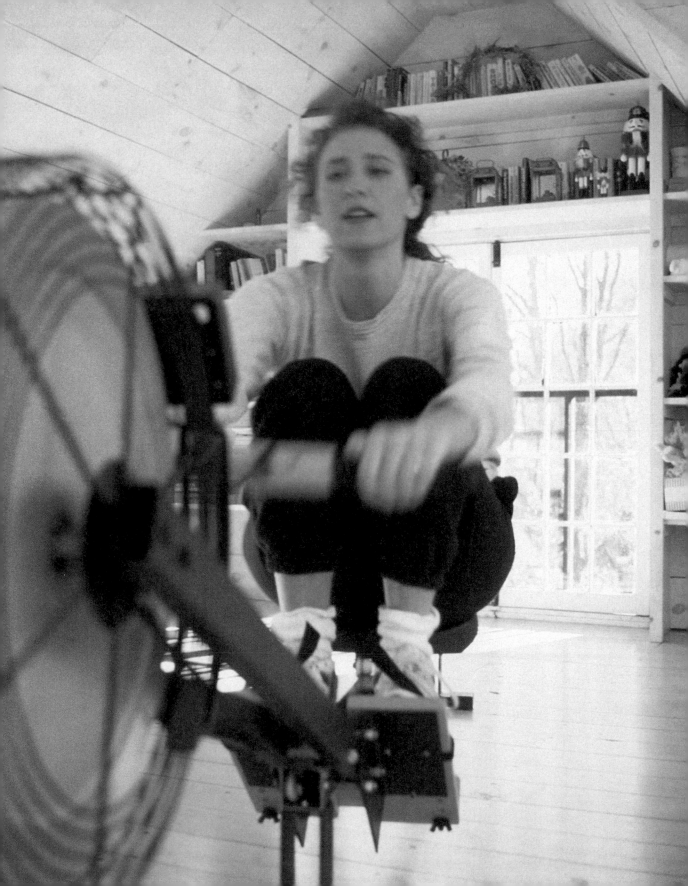

Chapter 12

Exercise (Your) Options

IT'S ALL WELL AND GOOD for me to say you should exercise more. But what should you do? How should you do it? Where and when and how often? Those are the questions this chapter will answer. Choosing the right exercise means developing a balanced weekly activity routine that suits your lifestyle, circumstances, preferences, and abilities.

In this chapter...

✓ The right exercise for you

✓ Think about your goals

✓ How will you do it?

✓ Are you a gym fan or a homebody?

✓ Balance your workout

✓ Make your choices

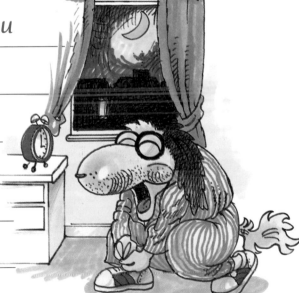

EXERCISING AT HOME IS CONVENIENT, BUT YOU NEED TO BE SELF-MOTIVATED

The right exercise for you

PUTTING MORE ACTIVITY INTO YOUR LIFE *is a matter of taking it a step at a time. It's unrealistic and unsafe to expect to go from couch potato to weekend warrior in a day, a week, or even a month. If you start off with something that is beyond your level of fitness, the chances are great that you will become discouraged and stop.*

The wrong way

I have a friend who was a cross-country runner in high school. In the intervening 40 years, he's shifted his extracurricular activity to reading gourmet cookbooks and eating the results of his research. Every once in a while, he decides he really should get some exercise, so he laces up his running shoes and runs for a mile. He comes home panting and sweating, lamenting that a mile just seems a lot longer than it used to. And that's the end of running until the next time . . . a month or more down the road. What he is doing is both foolish and dangerous. But you know that.

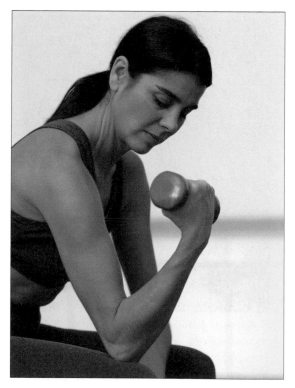

The right way

Another friend of mine had done little exercise for years when she decided she was looking pudgy and feeling low-energy. She joined a gym and started going to beginner-level exercise classes twice a week. On the days she did not take a class, she used the treadmill at 2 mph for 30 minutes and then did a training-machine circuit, using the lowest possible weights.

She told me that at first there were exercises she simply could not do. Double crunches, for example, put an impossible strain on her back. And there

■ **By starting slowly,** *using low weights and low-intensity aerobic exercise, you will gradually build up strength and stamina and tone up without overstraining your muscles.*

were others she could do, but not for as many reps as the instructor counted out. But she hung in there, doing as much as she could.

To her amazement and delight, she found she was gradually able to do more. As her abdominal muscles got stronger, so did her back. Double crunches were possible, though she still could not do as many as other people in the class. She increased her speed on the treadmill, getting up to 3 mph at a slight incline. She increased the weights on the training machines. Before long, she stopped feeling like the newest kid on the block. She did it the right way, and the results were obvious.

How fit are you? (revisited)

Take out your weight-loss notebook and turn to the part of your personal database that you filled out while doing the self-assessment in Chapter 8. Review your answers to the lifestyle activity quiz. If anything has changed, revise it.

If it's been a while since you filled out this section, take the strength, endurance, and flexibility yardstick tests again, and enter any changes into your database. If you took one of the online fitness tests, you might want to do it again, and enter any changes in your database.

The entries you now have in your personal database are what experts call your baseline, where you were when you began. As you become more active, you will be able to measure yourself against this baseline and see how much your fitness level has improved.

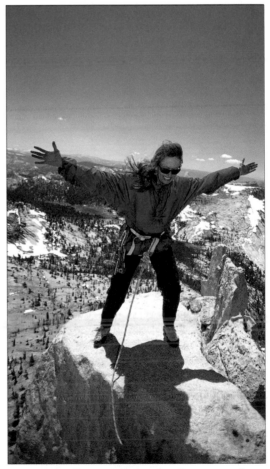

Your fitness level will improve as you begin to exercise more.

What seems to be just too hard may become just hard enough. And in time, what's hard enough will seem easy.

■ **As your fitness improves,** *the range of exercise options will broaden. You may find yourself getting involved in an adventure sport you wouldn't have dreamed of taking up before.*

Think about your goals

ACCORDING TO THE EXPERTS, *a universal goal should be 30 minutes of physical activity of moderate* **intensity** *on most days of the week. There's nothing that says you can't do more. And in the beginning, you may do less.*

The good news is that several short periods are as good as a single longer period, so long as it adds up to at least 30 minutes. That means if you have the time, or the endurance, for only 10 minutes at a time, you can get your daily dose in three sessions. For example, you could do some calisthenics in the morning, take a brisk but brief walk at lunch time, and play a quick game of tag with your kids just before dinner.

Take it a step at a time

Goals are excellent motivators, but they work best if you set both long-term and short-term ones. If you have been only somewhat active and want to be very active, you may get discouraged long before you reach that goal. If, on the other hand, you decide you'd like to increase the number of days in which you engage in physical activity from one a week to three a week by the end of next month, that is a reasonable goal.

Breaking up your goals into smaller chunks is even more reasonable. You might begin by adding 10 minutes to each activity period. When you are up to 30 minutes on each day you exercise, you can add another day.

Intensity can be measured by how hard your heart works during any activity. The faster your heart rate, the more intense the activity. That makes intensity a relative term: What is moderately intense for you might be only minimally intense for someone who is very fit, and extremely intense for someone who is less fit than you are. Think of minimal intensity as the lower end of your target heart rate (THR) zone, high intensity as the upper end, and moderate intensity as the area in between. Check your THR zone on your personal database.

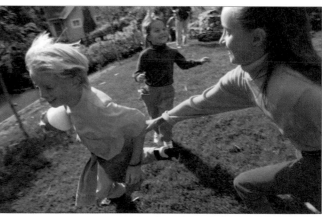

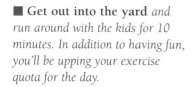

■ **Get out into the yard** *and run around with the kids for 10 minutes. In addition to having fun, you'll be upping your exercise quota for the day.*

The same goes for the fitness yardsticks. Set a long term goal, but break it into a series of short-term ones.

Can you do five more jumping jacks and still stay in your THR zone? Once you can do five more, aim for ten. Can you do five more sit-ups before your abdominal muscles tire and you start losing perfect form? Then aim for ten more. Can you increase your reach by 2 inches? Aim for 4 inches.

If you took one of the online fitness tests, you might want to set a long-term and several short-term goals for bettering your fitness score.

If you are extremely overweight, don't attempt to sweat off the pounds in a week. If you've been a couch potato, don't start training for the marathon. If you're somewhat active, gradually increase the frequency of your activities, but don't overdo it. If you're moderately active, try to increase the intensity of your activities or try something new. In all cases, choose activities that are appropriate for your current level of fitness.

Do not choose any physical activity for which you are not fit. At best, you won't be able to keep it up. At worst, you will injure yourself.

INHALE/EXHALE

If your idea of exerting yourself includes taking a deep breath and then holding it while you push, pull, or lift, have I got news for you! You'll get a lot more mileage if you exhale forcefully on the effort. Of course, that requires you to inhale deeply just before the effort.

Whether you are doing sit-ups, lifting weights, whacking a tennis ball, or just reaching for your toes, start with an inhale and then blow out as you do the work.

How will you do it?

I LIVE NEAR A BEAUTIFUL PARK with a measured
*running track. The park is filled at all hours with what looks like
a companionable crowd happily jogging their way to
fitness. Sometimes I have fantasies about joining them.*

But the truth is I hate jogging. It rattles my bones. It hurts my
feet, my ankles, my shins. I quickly get out of breath. And I
find it boring. If someone told me that the only way I could
get and stay fit was to become a runner, I think I'd sit down
on the curb and give up.

Lucky for me – and for you – there are dozens of ways to be
active. No one has to choose a way that is unpleasant, painful,
or unsuitable from the point of view of fitness. The trick is to
find activities that you like and that you can do.

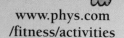

INTERNET

**www.phys.com
/fitness/activities**

*If you're still not sure where
to begin, click on "Sports &
Activities" for details on
more than two dozen popular
choices. You'll find out
what's involved and tips on
how to get started.*

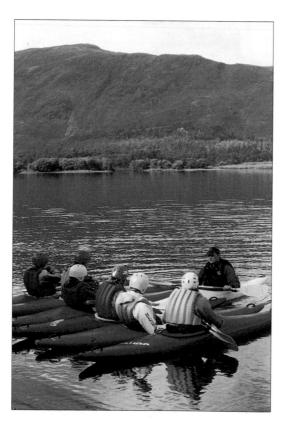

The reason I know about that running track
is that I often ride a bike nearby. For me,
bike riding is ideal. I can travel through
pleasant surroundings, as fast or slow as
I please. My leg muscles are working hard
without stressing my joints. When I pedal
fast or uphill, I work up quite a sweat. And
I do a lot of deep breathing. I can definitely
get an aerobic workout on my bike.

Bike riding is not the only thing I do.
It is not an all-round activity. It does
not strengthen my back and abdominal
muscles, nor do much for my arms. It's easy
on my joints, but doesn't really increase my
flexibility. And in the climate where I live,
it is definitely not a four-season activity.
That's why I joined a gym.

■ **Getting fit is enjoyable** *when you're involved
in an activity that you love. From canoeing to
horseback riding, mountain biking to golfing, you
can choose from dozens of ways to be active.*

An exercise grab bag

Short on ideas about what you can do? Here's a list of physical activities, ranging from mild and moderate to heavy-duty. I bet you can find a handful that will appeal to you.

- Aerobics: low impact, high impact, step
- Baseball
- Basketball
- Bicycling: stationary, racing, touring, mountain biking
- Bowling
- Boxing
- Calisthenics
- Canoeing
- Dancing: ballet, ballroom, salsa, disco, tap
- Dog walking
- Fencing
- Frisbee
- Football: touch, full contact
- Gardening
- Gymnastics
- Golf
- Handball
- Hiking
- Hockey
- Housework
- Ice skating
- Jogging
- Judo
- Jumping rope
- Kayaking
- Lawn mowing
- Martial arts: judo, karate, tae kwon do, t'ai chi, kickboxing
- Orienteering
- Paddleball
- Power yoga
- Racewalking
- Racquetball
- Rapelling
- Rock climbing
- Rowing

- Running
- Scuba diving
- Skating
- Skateboarding
- Skiing: downhill, cross country
- Snowshoeing
- Soccer
- Squash
- Stair climbing
- Stretching
- Swimming
- Tennis
- Volleyball
- Walking
- Yard work
- Yoga

Did I leave anything out?

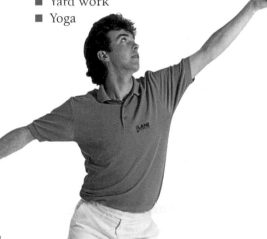

■ **Tennis** *is great for raising fitness levels and, being a sociable game, is ideal for those who don't like to work out alone.*

Don't forget to stretch

Stretching is important for everyone, but it is particularly important for beginners.

Gently warm up and stretch the muscles you will be using before you begin any kind of activity.

If you're a beginner

If the last time you did a jumping jack was in high school gym class, start slowly. Your body is not used to working hard. Your muscles are probably quite weak and your ligaments fairly stiff. You may not know how to breathe effectively. All of these things will improve in time, but give yourself a chance to get used to being more active.

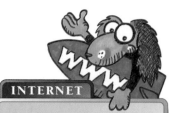

INTERNET

www.phys.com /fitness/stretches

Want to know more about stretching? The "Stretching Guide" at this web site will tell you why and when to do it. Keep clicking and you'll see exactly how to do enough stretches to keep you supple for life.

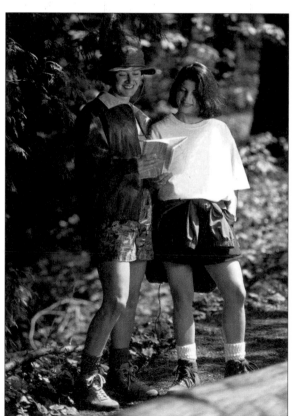

Walking is a good way for beginners to begin. It is second nature to most of us. It's really just a matter of doing it more and more often. Walking for as little as 30 minutes a day can make a big difference to your health and fitness.

■ **Put on a pair** *of comfortable and supportive shoes, some nonrestrictive clothing and set out to cover some ground. You may find your outing more enjoyable if you go with a friend.*

When I say "walking," don't think walking up to the corner to buy a loaf of bread or ambling through the park. I am talking about setting off deliberately to cover some ground.

Begin by setting a time limit. Walk for 15 minutes or a half hour. Keep up an even pace. Try to take a route that has both flat ground and some gentle inclines. Move your arms as well as your legs. And breathe!

One of the nicest things about walking is that you can vary your route. That keeps it from being boring. You may also find it easier if you do it with a friend or clamp on some headphones and listen to music while you walk.

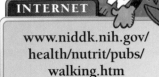

INTERNET

www.niddk.nih.gov/ health/nutrit/pubs/ walking.htm

The National Institute of Diabetes and Digestive and Kidney Diseases has a terrific publication, available online, called "Walking . . . A Step in the Right Direction," with all the whys and hows of starting a walking program.

If you're somewhat to moderately active

People who are somewhat to moderately active have many more choices than card-carrying couch potatoes. Your challenge is to move to the next level. You can do that by adding minutes of activity to each day or adding days of activity to your week. You can up the intensity or try something new. The important thing is to be sure you push yourself a bit, or involve yourself in exercise groups or settings that will do the pushing for you.

One way to challenge yourself is to focus on your THR, aiming for several weekly sessions in which you push yourself into the upper range for 20 to 30 minutes.

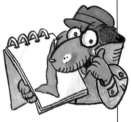

Aerobic exercise is the key here. Running, dancing, step aerobics, and kick boxing are among the many possible choices.

DEFINITION

Interval training *is a way of intensifying an aerobic workout by increasing speed to increase heart rate in measured bursts. Typically, the greater intensity is maintained for a full minute every 3 to 5 minutes during the workout.*

Interval training is another way to give yourself a push. Punctuate an aerobics session with short "power bursts" – 1 minute of greater speed or intensity every 3 to 5 minutes.

213

Still another way to challenge yourself is to work on building your strength. Lifting progressively heavier weights or increasing the number of *reps* or *sets* will pay off in firmer and stronger muscles. Whatever you do, drink lots of water.

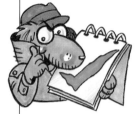

Keep a plastic bottle half filled with water in your freezer. Top it off and take it with you whenever you set off for an activity. If you don't like the icy feel of it, slip the bottle into a gym sock.

Even if you don't think you're sweating, you'll need extra water when you exercise. Working your muscles produces lactic acid, a toxin that causes muscle fatigue. The only way to flush it out is with water.

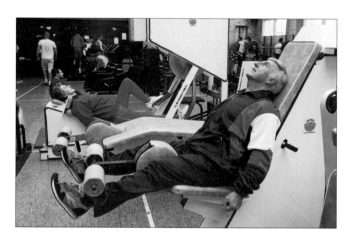

■ **Once you can manage** *a certain weight or number of repetitions comfortably, don't stop there. Keep setting yourself new, more ambitious targets to improve your strength.*

If you have special needs

If you are extremely overweight, over 65, pregnant, disabled, or have a chronic disease, choosing a more active lifestyle is more complicated than simply deciding what you like to do and just doing it.

That does not mean you shouldn't even think about exercise. It does mean you should get advice before you make any changes.

If there are medical restrictions on how active you can be, talk to your doctor about what you can and cannot do.

You may be surprised to discover that some of these restrictions are imaginary.

You may have to take it slowly. You will certainly have to choose activities that are possible for you and do not add stress to the parts of your body affected by your condition. There may be special strategies or precautions you will have to take. But be assured that even baby steps will get you closer to your goals. And don't forget to give yourself a big pat on the back, every day, for trying the best you can.

Are you a gym fan or a homebody?

INTERNET

www.drkoop.com /wellness/fitness

There are so many special situations and the limitations put on physical activity vary so widely that making specific recommendations is not practical. Instead, I recommend the "Exercise with Care" section of the Fitness Center on this web site. It features discussions of exercise for everyone from people with asthma and arthritis to those who use wheelchairs.

SOME PEOPLE LIKE TO EXERCISE *alone and others would rather do it with a friend or even a crowd. There is no particular advantage to either. What's important is that you know what you prefer. If turning up at an exercise class in a pair of shorts makes you want to crawl back under the covers, wear those shorts and exercise at home. If, on the other hand, a regular date to go for a run with a friend is what gets you up and moving, that's the choice for you.*

Join the crowd

If you like to exercise with others, join a gym or health club, sign up for classes, make an ironclad appointment with a friend or family member.

Committing time and/or money, especially when someone else is involved, may be the key to making sure you actually get up and do it.

Team and competitive sports are also ways to make physical activity fun. This works best for people who are motivated by competition. A weekly volleyball or softball game may be just the ticket.

INTERNET

www.prevention.com /weight/quiz

"What's Your Workout Personality" is the question this quiz helps you answer. It asks ten questions (which have nothing to do with fitness or activity) and then recommends a form of exercise to suit your personal style.

IS THIS GYM FOR YOU?

There are a lot of gyms and health clubs that charge a lot of money, have glossy clientele, and have all the warmth and coziness of a singles bar on Saturday night. If you are out of shape and lumpy, the thought of joining one of these may put an end to your exercise plans. I don't blame you.

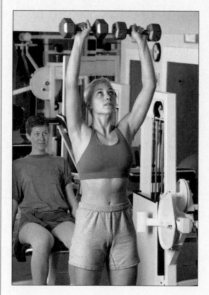

They are not, however, your only option. For example, I belong to a low-cost "women only" gym that is short on frills and long on sisterhood. Members come in all colors, ages, shapes, and degree of "buffness." It is a comfortable place to which I am enormously loyal. Ys and other community centers often have exercise programs, some of them divided by gender, age, and skill level.

If you feel intimidated by the "scene" at a particular health club, look for one that fits your personality better.

■ **If you enjoy** *working out with other people around you and you like using exercise machines, joining a gym is probably the way to go.*

If there's a running club in your vicinity, you might want to give it a try. Many such clubs have sections for beginners, so you won't find yourself panting behind the world-class sprinters.

There are many ways to be active that aren't "athletic." Do you feel like dancing? From ballroom to disco, ballet to jazz, you'll get a good aerobic workout and have fun while you're doing it. Combining an evening's entertainment with your daily dose of exercise may be the smartest thing you do all weekend.

If you prefer to exercise alone

There's nothing wrong with exercising alone, as long as you really do it. Set aside a specific time each day and keep your appointment with yourself. If you work out at home, put on your exercise garb, clear enough space on the floor, and unplug the phone. This is your time, so don't let yourself be interrupted. You might want to pop an exercise video into your VCR or tune into one of the many exercise programs on cable television. If you do your own routine, be sure to play some music to help you keep up a lively pace.

Should you invest in home exercise equipment? In my opinion, treadmills, steppers, ski trackers, weight machines, and ab conditioners are notorious dust collectors. The good ones are expensive and the bargain ones are flimsy. Most are single-purpose gadgets, which will bore you before they earn their keep.

If you like exercising with machines, joining a gym is a better bet.

Most gyms have a wide variety of heavy-duty machines, and you don't have to worry about keeping them dust-free and in working condition.

Just because you like to exercise alone doesn't mean you have to stay home. Swimming is basically a solitary pursuit, but an excellent workout for those who like it. Running can be done solo as well as with one or more partners.

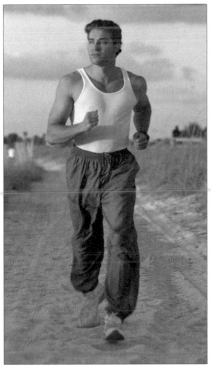

■ **If you choose** *to exercise alone, be sure to monitor your motivators. Doing it is up to you. No one else will know if you've taken the day off.*

Balance your workout

BE SURE TO BUILD VARIETY *into your choices of exercise. One of the biggest mistakes you can make is to do the same thing day after day. Not only will you get bored, and then stop doing it, but your body needs a chance to rest and restore itself.*

In general, exercise can be divided between aerobic and resistance, also called anaerobic, activities. To keep it simple, aerobic exercise makes you breathe hard and elevates your heart rate. Resistance exercise involves lifting, pushing, or pulling against some kind of weight. This increases muscle strength. The most common example of resistance exercise is strength or weight training.

Whatever activities you choose, be sure to pick some from column A (anaerobic exercise) and some from column B (aerobic exercise).

The best thing is to alternate between anaerobic and aerobic types of activity.

It is especially important to give yourself a day or two off between resistance-training sessions. Your muscles need to recover from the workout. On your off days, try some aerobic exercise. A balanced routine would involve, for example, a day of strength training, followed by a day of swimming; you could go back to weights or calisthenics the following day, and take a bike ride the day after. Another day of strength training could be followed by dancing. You get the idea.

Don't forget to warm up and cool down. Cold muscles are prone to injury, so get your blood flowing before you exert them. Run in place, do some knee bends, swing your arms, rotate your pelvis. And don't stop cold after you've worked up a sweat. Slow down and lower the intensity of whatever you're doing, then gradually come to a stop.

Exercise with the seasons

Use the special qualities of the seasons where you live to add spice to your activities. Skiing, snowboarding, and ice skating are wonderful ways to be active in the winter. Don't let rain be an excuse to take the day off; that's a good time to go to the gym. If you're prone to allergies, plan indoor alternatives during allergy season. If the summer heat makes you feel listless, dive into the pool and swim some laps. And don't let a beautiful fall day pass you by – get out and do something!

DEFINITION

Anaerobic *means without oxygen. That does not mean you shouldn't breathe while doing this kind of exercise. What it does mean is that this type of physical effort emphasizes muscle building rather than cardiovascular fitness. Resistance training – pushing or pulling against a weight or other opposing force – is anaerobic exercise. Running, jumping, swimming, and dancing are examples of aerobic exercise.*

INTERNET

www.prevention.com/ weight/planner

This web site has an extensive menu of workouts that you can mix and match to fit your goals and preferences.

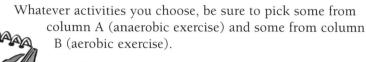

■ **Skiing is a great** *way to keep yourself active in winter, especially if you live within easy distance of mountains and snow.*

Make your choices

TAKE OUT YOUR WEIGHT-LOSS NOTEBOOK *and make a list of activities you'd like to try. You might want to organize them under these headings:*

- Do These Now
- Do These When I'm More Fit
- Do These Indoors
- Do These Outdoors
- Do These Alone

- Do These with Others
- Do These in Winter
- Do These in Spring
- Do These in Summer
- Do These in Fall

Keep this list handy whenever you have the urge to do something active, and especially when you don't. If you think of it as a menu, it may whet your appetite to get up and moving.

A simple summary

✓ Choose physical activities suited to your own level of fitness.

✓ Don't overdo it. Gradually increase the level of your activity, taking it a step at a time.

✓ The more regularly you exercise, the more fit you will become.

✓ Increase the time and intensity of your activities as your fitness level improves.

✓ Long-term fitness goals will keep you motivated; short-term goals will keep you on track.

✓ If you are extremely overweight, over 65, pregnant, disabled, or have a chronic disease, talk to your doctor before beginning any new activity.

✓ When, where, and how you exercise should suit your personality and preferences.

✓ Your workout must be balanced and varied to ensure that it is safe, challenging, and interesting.

✓ Keep a list of activities you like in your weight-loss notebook to motivate you all year round.

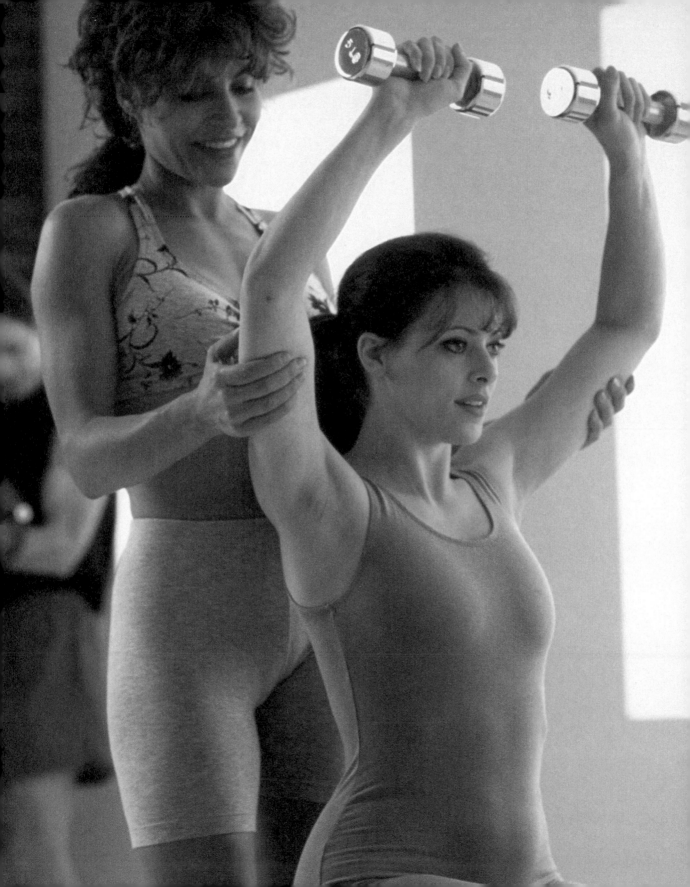

Chapter 13

Get Advice, Get Ideas

THERE IS NO SINGLE DIET and exercise plan that is right for everyone. The food you eat and the kind of exercise you do are based on personal preferences. Still, it's a good idea to do some research and get as much information as is practical before you decide how you will go about losing weight. There are many sources of advice and ideas, some more reliable than others. Here's how to tell which to trust and which to take with a grain of salt or avoid altogether.

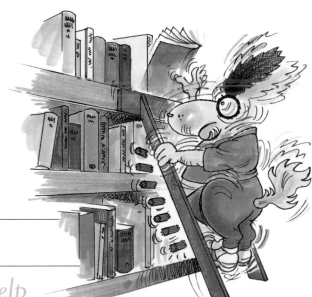

In this chapter...

✓ Talk to the pros

✓ Media messages

✓ If you need some help

YOU DON'T HAVE TO GO IT ALONE: PERSONAL TRAINERS AND OTHER PROFESSIONALS CAN HELP

Talk to the pros

THE BEST PLACE TO BEGIN is with professionals, people who are educated and trained in health and nutrition. Although it is a good idea for anyone who wants to lose weight, consulting a professional is a must for certain people: those with chronic illnesses, teenagers, the elderly, and pregnant women.

Start with your doctor

I have already suggested talking with your doctor. Ideally, he or she knows the latest on the health risks of overweight and will be able to evaluate your particular risks. Doctors may not be the best source of information about effective strategies for losing weight, however.

Give your doctor a chance to show that he or she can be a strong partner in your weight-loss effort. Bring up the topic, if it has not been raised already, and discuss it fully. Bring along your weight-loss notebook.

Your food and activity diaries will be particularly useful when you discuss your eating and exercise habits with your doctor and look at what needs to change.

Here are some questions to explore:

a Are you overweight?

b If so, by how much?

c Do you have weight-related health problems?

d How much can you reasonably expect to lose over the course of how much time?

e Are there specific foods or types of food you should avoid or be certain to eat?

f Are there any limitations on the type and amount of exercise you can do?

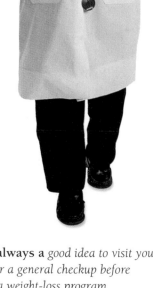

■ **It is always a** *good idea to visit your doctor for a general checkup before starting a weight-loss program.*

g What sorts of problems have you had in the past when you tried to lose weight?

h Are these problems mostly behavioral?

i What specific advice and strategies can your doctor suggest?

Talk to other specialists

If you are not getting the kind of advice you need from your doctor, say so. Emphasize how important it is to you to get the time and attention you need on this subject. If you are still not satisfied, ask for a referral to another professional who will be able to help. Don't get frustrated if your doctor is not able or willing to help. Give it a reasonable try and then move on – to a different doctor or to a different type of professional.

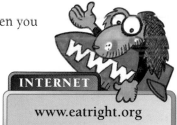

INTERNET

www.eatright.org

The American Dietetic Association web site is a good place to learn about what dietitians do. You can also use it to find a registered dietitian in your area.

DEFINITION

Nutritionist *is a general term for someone who gives advice about food and nutrition. Anyone can claim to be a nutritionist since it does not require or even imply specialized education or licensing.* **Dietitians** *have college-level and sometimes graduate-level education in nutrition science and are licensed by the American Dietetic Association (ADA). ADA offers two credentials: registered dietitian (RD), which requires a bachelor's degree, and dietetic technician, registered (DTR), which requires a 2-year associate's degree. Clinical nutritionists have doctoral-level training (MD or PhD).*

If your doctor cannot make a referral, check with your employer, health plan, or local medical society. If there is a hospital in your area, ask if it has a weight-loss clinic or a staff *nutritionist* or *dietitian*.

If you consult a nutritionist or dietitian you don't know, be sure to ask about the person's professional credentials. Look for practitioners who are members of either the American Dietetic Association and the American Society for Clinical Nutrition.

Be wary of anyone who wants to sell you a "diet plan" or special supplements.

223

PERSONAL TRAINERS

Personal trainers are like private exercise tutors. They custom design an exercise routine for you, show you how to do the moves, and push you to really work out. You pay by the session, and the price can really add up.

For some people, this is money well spent. For others, it is out of the question.

If you'd like to give it a try, consider hiring a personal trainer for one or two sessions, and then take it from there yourself. Or you could have one or a few training sessions and then a "booster" session every month or so.

Most gyms and health clubs have personal trainers on staff or can refer you to one. Be sure you work with someone who is trained and certified. There are a number of certification associations, but one of the most reputable is the American Council on Exercise. Visit their web site to find out more about personal trainers in general, and their certification standards in particular.

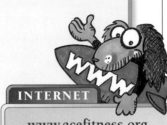

INTERNET

www.acefitness.org

The American Council on Exercise web site is full of information on fitness. You can also find the name and contact information for ACE-certified personal trainers by city or zip code.

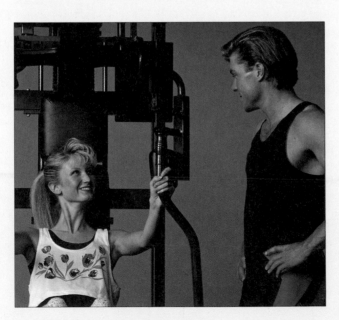

■ **Personal trainers** *will study your exercise capabilities, and give you a workout that will complement your diet.*

Media messages

BOOKS, MAGAZINES, TELEVISION, radio, and the Internet are loaded – to tell the truth, they're overloaded – with information and ideas about weight loss. Used intelligently, they can be helpful. But take care not to be overwhelmed or misled.

Read all about it

Browse the diet/nutrition and exercise/fitness shelves of your local bookstore for ideas. You do not have to swallow whole any single book, but you may be able to gather enough ideas and information from several of them to help you formulate your own weight-loss plan.

Don't believe everything you read in diet books.

When you look at diet books, remember what we talked about in Chapter 10. You will face a barrage of fad diets, but I've given you the ammo to defend yourself. Diet cookbooks are an excellent source of ideas. I hope you'll be doing more home cooking, since that's the best way to control what goes into your mouth. And even if you don't have diabetes, cookbooks intended for people with this disease tend to emphasize the same sensible eating principles that lead to weight loss.

Magazines are another source of diet ideas. Your choices include women's magazines (men can read them too), sports and fitness magazines, and magazines devoted entirely to diet. As with books, don't believe everything you read. Because they have to come up with "hot new" ideas for every issue, magazines are even more likely than books to feature fad diets. Many of them present digested versions of the latest best-selling diet book or exercise trend.

Magazines work best as mini-motivators for short-term goals. If you're wondering how to get started, these may be a good bet.

INTERNET

diabetes.org

You don't have to have diabetes to take advantage of the many good ideas at the web site of the American Diabetes Association. Click on the "Recipe of the Day" and "Tips for Healthy Eating."

INTERNET

magazine-rack.com

Many magazines have their own web sites, so you can check out articles that interest you without having to buy the entire issue or read articles in back issues that you may have missed. Use your favorite search engine or click on this web site for a large selection of online magazines organized by subject.

Click with care

Search "weight loss" on the Internet and you will find enough sites to keep you busy for a year. The www boxes throughout this book will lead you to some of them and many of those will, in turn, link you to others. Don't believe everything you click on. Setting up a web site is cheap and easy. Anyone can do it.

Avoid sites that ask you to pay for their advice or that are selling specific weight-loss aids and other products.

Be sure you can tell the difference between one person's opinion or experience shared in a chat group; solid, verifiable medical or scientific information; and advertising hype.

Stick with sources you can identify and know are reliable. For example:

a) Government web sites from the Food and Drug Administration, U.S. Department of Agriculture, and such members of the National Institutes of Health as the National Institute of Diabetes and Digestive and Kidney Diseases and the National Heart, Lung, and Blood Institute.

b) Web sites that are maintained by hospital-based, weight-loss clinics, medical organizations, and foundations devoted to specific diseases and conditions.

c) Web sites from reputable publications, ranging from medical journals and health and nutrition newsletters to respected consumer magazines.

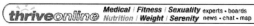

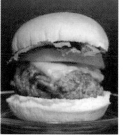

thriveonline Medical | Fitness | Sexuality experts · boards   Nutrition | Weight | Serenity news · chat · map   **Newsletters** Eight ways to thrive

healthy dieting guidelines
by joan salge blake, m.s., r.d.

IS YOUR DIET HARMING YOUR HEART?

arch-enemy, artery-clotting saturated fat should be kept, on average, to less than 10 percent of your total calories daily. Ideally, your total fat intake (including mono- and poly-unsaturated fats) should be harnessed to no more than 30 percent of your daily calories. Saturated fat is predominately from animal sources, such as fatty cuts of meat and whole-milk dairy products. Choosing lean meats, skinless poultry, and low-fat or nonfat dairy products will help put a cap on saturated fat.

back to: dieting guidelines main page
see also: nutrition main page

Yes, some things are too good to be true. If your plan allows cheesy burgers, your arteries will suffer in the long run (even if you drop pounds in the meantime).

■ **Web sites** *about dieting and weight loss abound, many of them offering sound advice. Just make sure you know the difference between fact and hype.*

INTERNET

usda.gov/cnpp

niddk.nih.gov

nhlbi.nih.gov/health/pubs

Visit the web sites of the Center for Nutrition Policy and Promotion, the National Institute of Diabetes and Digestive and Kidney Diseases, and the National Heart, Lung, and Blood Institute for solid information on diet and exercise and useful links.

If you need some help

LOSING WEIGHT BY YOURSELF *may suit your personality and temperament. Or you may do better with some company and some help. The simplest way to decide which is the case is to look back at your weight-loss notebook. Reread your answers to the "What Food Means to Me" quiz as well as your essay about your hopes and fears.*

If you have been on many diets and not succeeded in losing weight or keeping it off, a team approach may make sense for you.

Your choices for your diet range from a structured weight-loss program to formal support groups and diet buddies.

Structured weight-loss systems

These are for-profit commercial ventures that promote their own weight-loss philosophy and, in many cases, sell prepackaged foods and meal replacement products. Some of the better known programs are Weight Watchers, Jenny Craig, Nutri/System, the Diet Center, and the Cambridge Diet. They all have web sites and are listed in your local phone directory.

I do not intend to recommend or to discourage you from investigating any or all of these. Instead, I will offer some guidelines to help you evaluate what they offer. Most structured diet plans tend to dictate specific foods you can eat. There are both pros and cons to this approach.

- **The pros:** On the plus side, the more rigid a plan's requirement, the less likely you will accidentally eat the wrong thing. And if you do, you will know you are cheating. For some people, this is helpful. Only you know if you're such a person.

- **The cons:** The problem with a rigid diet is that you may be unable to stick to it for long. For one thing, it gets boring very fast. For another, it limits you when someone else is doing the menu planning: at parties, restaurants, and even within your own household.

In addition, some, but not all, structured plans include physical activity and behavior modification in their program.

INTERNET

www.thriveonline.com

Click on "Weight Management" and then "Programs & Products" for the lowdown on all of the commercial weight-loss programs.

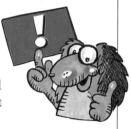

Weight-loss plans that focus only on what you eat will not be lastingly effective.

Remember: To make your weight loss last, you need to eat in a different way for the rest of your life. Take a look at how any plan promises to deal with weight maintenance. The maintenance phase is even more important than the weight-loss phase. Can you keep it up? Will you want to?

These plans also cost money. Again, there are two sides to this coin. You can certainly lose weight without paying anyone to help you. And the cost does add up over time. On the other hand, you may be more motivated to stick with it if you are sinking your hard-earned dough into your weight-loss efforts.

Support groups

Some of the commercial weight-loss programs may offer group counseling and support groups, but such programs are not the only source of emotional support for dieters. Many Ys, community centers, churches and other houses of worship also sponsor support groups. There are even online communities that provide an opportunity for hopeful weight losers to bolster each other's efforts.

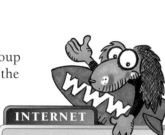

INTERNET

www.overeaters anonymous.org

You can find general information about Overeaters Anonymous on this web site as well as the location of a chapter near you. There's also a quiz: "15 questions to help you determine if you are an overeater."

a **Overeaters Anonymous (OA):** This nonprofit organization has affiliates in many towns and cities. Modeled on the 12-step approach that originated with Alcoholics Anonymous, Overeaters Anonymous brings together people with food and eating behavior problems, who help each other conquer compulsive eating. OA does not espouse a particular diet or weight-loss philosophy, although it does focus on compulsive eating. If your weight problem does not involve compulsive eating, OA may not be for you.

INTERNET

www.tops.org

The web site of Take Off Pounds Sensibly (TOPS®) will tell you how to sign up for this program and give you a lot of information about its philosophy and approach to weight loss.

b **Take Off Pounds Sensibly (TOPS®):** TOPS® is another nonprofit diet and support group, but unlike OA it charges annual membership dues. It combines group educational and support meetings with a sensible and nutritionally balanced diet.

QUESTIONS TO ASK ABOUT STRUCTURED DIET PLANS

Before you hand over a penny, ask these questions about the weight-loss plan you are considering:

1. Do I have to sign a contract to participate in the plan? If so, what does the fine print say?

2. Is there a trial period or other escape clause if I decide it's not for me after I have signed up?

3. Will I receive an individualized assessment of my weight and realistic weight-loss goals before beginning the program? Is there any additional fee for this?

4. Is group or individual counseling included in the plan? Is there any additional fee for this?

5. What are the professional qualifications and credentials of personnel?

6. What is the schedule for meetings and appointments? Is it compatible with my own schedule?

7. How many calories per day will the plan's diet allow me?

8. Is the recommended diet nutritionally balanced?

9. Does the weight-loss program include exercise and other physical activity?

10. Is there a maintenance and follow-up program? If so, is there an additional charge for this?

11. Will I be required to buy special nutritional formulas or supplements? If so, what do they cost? What are the ingredients?

12. Are there any other hidden costs or conditions of membership?

13. Are there any known health risks for those following the plan?

- **Weight-loss chat groups:** The World Wide Web is the home of chat groups and message boards on every subject imaginable, including weight loss. Because these involve just plain folks talking to other folks, the advice offered must be taken with a grain of salt. Nonetheless, you may find it enormously helpful to exchange ideas, frustrations, and information with people who are in the same boat as you. Use your favorite search engine to find online weight-loss chat groups.

- **Closer to home:** Don't forget your own friends and family. Look back at your weight-loss notebook and the list you made of "Friends of My Diet." These people can be your support group, and there may even be one or more people on that list who would be happy to join you on your climb.

Other things that may help

You may benefit from one or more of a variety of techniques to help you deal with emotional, spiritual, and physical hunger. Psychotherapy may be helpful for people who can trace their overweight to emotional issues. This is especially important for people who are depressed or who suffer from eating disorders.

As with the weight-loss programs, money is involved in all of these approaches. If you're interested in exploring any of them, try one for a short while. See whether the approach is indeed helpful and the investment increases your motivation or whether you decide that the cost outweighs the benefit you are receiving.

INTERNET

www.thriveonline.com/ message_boards/

Among the message boards on this site is one on diet plans, programs, and products. Click on "Weight" to zero in on any diet or plan you are curious about, from the Atkins and Beverly Hills diets to Herbalife and the Zone.

- **Alternative therapeutic** *techniques such as hypnosis, acupuncture, and acupressure have helped some people in their weight-loss efforts.*

Read your weight-loss diary

One of the best sources of ideas is the book you are writing yourself. Your food and activity diaries are full of information about your eating and exercise habits. The entries in your Personal Database will tell you where you are now. Your list of long- and short-term goals outlines clearly where you want to go. Your menu of exercise options contains clues about how to get there.

Spend some time studying your notes to prepare yourself for the task in the next chapter: designing the diet and exercise program that will work for you.

A simple summary

✓ Before you begin to change the way you eat and exercise, get advice from your doctor and other professionals.

✓ If you are pregnant, over 65 years of age, suffer from a chronic disease or disabling condition, do not even think about changing the way you eat and exercise without first discussing it with your doctor.

✓ Before you begin to change the way you eat and exercise, get some ideas from books, magazines, the Internet, and other sources of information.

✓ Use what you know about nutrition, metabolism, physical activity, and weight loss to evaluate any of the advice and information you get.

✓ Structured weight-loss programs may be helpful, but be sure to research them and analyze the pros and cons before you sign on.

✓ Working with a personal trainer may well be helpful, but do give it a try before you commit yourself to a major investment of time and money.

✓ Support is available from many sources. Find the ones that will work for you if you don't want to go it alone.

✓ Your weight-loss notebook contains information about where you will go from here.

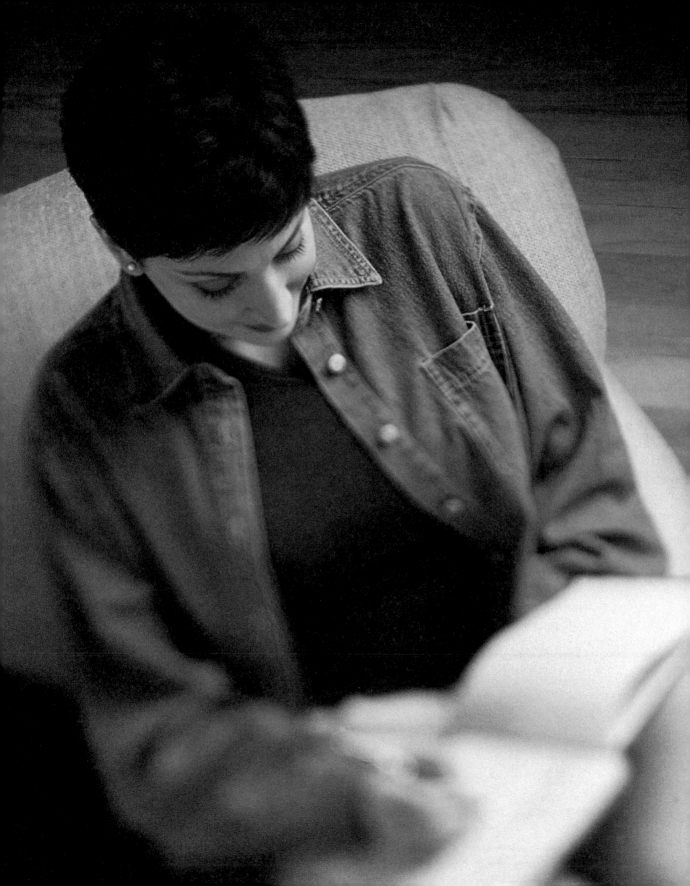

Chapter 14

This Is Your Weight-Loss Plan

OKAY, THIS IS IT! Time to design a daily plan for eating and exercise that will help you lose the weight you want to be rid of and begin a more active and healthy life style. The plan will be based on the principle of calories in–calories out. Think of the plan you will construct in this chapter as a first draft. Try it for a week and then reassess it. You may revise it once you have a better idea of what it's like to live with on a daily basis. Take out your weight-loss notebook and let's get started.

In this chapter...

✓ Apply what you know about yourself

✓ Plan your daily calorie expenditure

✓ Plan your daily calorie intake

✓ Write it all down

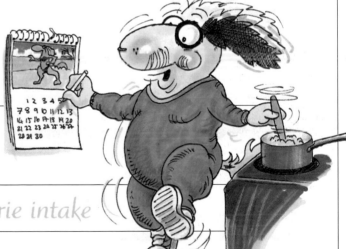

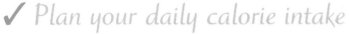

A WELL-PREPARED PLAN WILL GUIDE YOU TO SUCCESS

Apply what you know about yourself

WEIGHT LOSS IS NOT A ONE-SIZE-FITS-ALL AFFAIR. *It would be unfair, misleading, and ineffective if I told you how many calories you need to eliminate from your daily total to lose a predetermined amount of weight within a predetermined period of time. Fortunately, we can come pretty close to finding the size that fits you, now and in the future, when you are closer to the weight you consider ideal.*

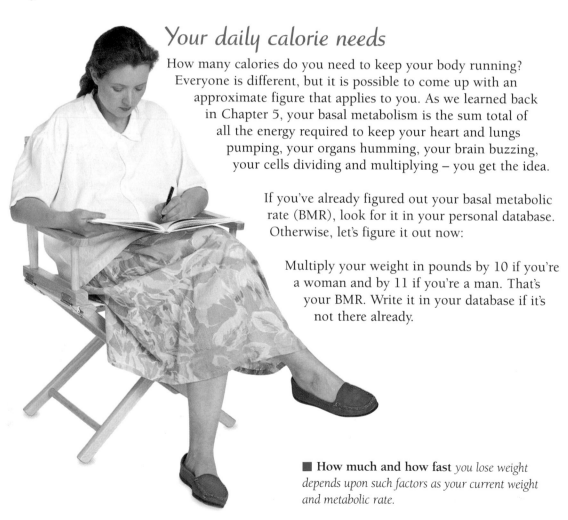

Your daily calorie needs

How many calories do you need to keep your body running? Everyone is different, but it is possible to come up with an approximate figure that applies to you. As we learned back in Chapter 5, your basal metabolism is the sum total of all the energy required to keep your heart and lungs pumping, your organs humming, your brain buzzing, your cells dividing and multiplying – you get the idea.

If you've already figured out your basal metabolic rate (BMR), look for it in your personal database. Otherwise, let's figure it out now:

Multiply your weight in pounds by 10 if you're a woman and by 11 if you're a man. That's your BMR. Write it in your database if it's not there already.

■ **How much and how fast** *you lose weight depends upon such factors as your current weight and metabolic rate.*

234

In addition to calories to run your body, you need some to fuel your activity. Look back at your personal database to find your activity level. If you didn't figure it out before – or if you have been more or less active recently – go back to Chapter 8 and take the Lifestyle Activity Quiz now.

Depending on your score, multiply your BMR by one of the following percentages:

Sedentary: 20 percent of BMR
Somewhat active: 30 percent of BMR
Moderately active: 40 percent of BMR
Very active: 50 percent of BMR

Now add that figure to your BMR.

For example, if you are a somewhat active 180-pound male:

$$180 \times 11 = 1,980 \quad 1,980 \times 30\% = 594 \quad 1,980 + 594 = 2,574.$$

If you consume 2,574 calories a day, your weight will remain the same. You will neither gain nor lose.

This is an approximate figure. The calorie total is an average; on any given day, you may eat more or less than that, but over the course of a week or so, that intake would keep your weight stable. The formula does not take your age into account. If you are middle-aged or older, your calorie needs will be lower than if you are a teenager or a young adult. You may also have thyroid or other metabolic issues that might affect your BMR. And, finally, you are a human being, not a robot, so the way your body uses energy may be different from the theoretical average person. Still, this is a close enough figure to work with.

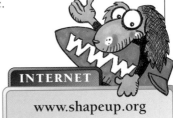

INTERNET

www.shapeup.org

Too much math? Go to the Cyberkitchen on this web site, and you can have your numbers crunched for you.

How much you need to subtract ✓

How much weight do you want to lose? Remember, every pound equals 3,500 calories. If you want to lose 5 pounds, that's 17,500 calories; 10 pounds would be 35,000; 20 would be 70,000, and so on. Write down your weight-loss goal and multiply by 3,500.

Now take a good hard look at that figure. If it's pretty big, think about losing it over an extended period of time. No matter how big it is, do not plan to lose it overnight.

Suppose you want to lose ten pounds. If you took only a month to do it, you'd have to reduce your daily calories by a little less than 1,200. Unless you are pigging out outrageously, 1,200 calories is a lot to eliminate in a single day.

Doing it over the course of two months would mean reducing daily calories by 500 to 600. Possible, but probably not easy. If you do it the way I recommend, you will not have to reduce the number of calories you eat by the whole amount.

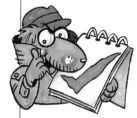

Losing weight will be easier and more effective if you combine eating less with exercising more.

For now, just take a stab at it. Divide your total calorie loss by 30, 60, 90 days or more, and then circle the option that looks reasonable to you. Label this "My daily calorie goal."

You may find it helpful to look back at your food diary. What was your weekly total calorie intake? Your weekly total expenditure? If you add between 500 and 1,000 calories to your weekly expenditure, how much would you have to subtract from what you eat? Divide that by 7. Do you think you can reduce your daily intake by that amount without feeling so deprived that you quit soon after you begin? Do you think you can add as little as 100 calories a day to your energy expenditure without feeling sore, bored, or pressed for time?

REMEMBER JANE DOE

The analysis I'm asking you to do is the same one Jane Doe did back in Chapter 9. You may want to reread the "What Jane planned" and "What Jane did" sidebars in that chapter, and see if the way she set her goals would work for you. If you sketched out a timetable at that time, look at it again. Does it still seem reasonable to you? Was it too ambitious? Not ambitious enough?

Write, or rewrite, a timetable like the one Jane made.

Here are some things to keep in mind:

- How far are you from your ideal weight?

- How far are you from a BMI in the healthy range?

- What are your long-term and short-term weight-loss goals?

- What holidays, seasons, vacations, weather, and other factors in the days ahead might make it easier or harder for you to stick to your plan?

What are your issues?

It may be easier to answer these questions if you think about the issues that have made you overweight to begin with. Look back at the answers you gave to "What food means to you."

1. Will you be able to make wiser food choices?

2. Will you be able to keep yourself from bingeing or otherwise violating your own rules?

3. Can you substitute some high-calorie foods with equally satisfying but lower-calorie choices?

4. Will you be able to avoid the triggers that make you eat more than you should?

5. Will you be able to enlist the help and support of the people around you?

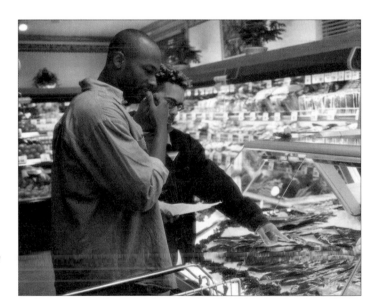

■ **To help you make** *the right food choices, make a list before you visit the store. Take a supportive friend along if you think you might be tempted to buy the wrong things, and don't go shopping on an empty stomach.*

Maybe getting enough exercise is more of a problem issue for you than food.

1. What is keeping you from being active?

2. Can you begin to include more exercise in your daily routine?

3. Can you manage to step up one rung on the lifestyle activity ladder?

Plan your daily calorie expenditure

YOU MAY BE WONDERING why I have put calories-out before calories-in. The short answer is: It's simpler that way.

Until you know how many calories you will be using, it's hard to figure out how many fewer you need to eat. So let's begin with your exercise routine and see how far that gets you toward your goal.

Planning for the plateau

There's another reason to focus on activity first. Call it the plateau, the set point, or whatever you like, as soon as you begin losing weight, your metabolic rate will go down and so will your calorie needs. If you started off as a 180-pound man with a BMR of 1,980, your BMR will be only 1,870 as soon as you become a 170-pound man. It will probably be even lower than that because your body, in its "wisdom," will have shifted into famine mode. However, when you were a 180-pound man, you gave yourself an extra 30 percent for being somewhat active. If you have added activity along with your diet, you may be able to make that an extra 40 percent which will raise your metabolic rate so you can, in fact, eat a few more calories. Here's the math:

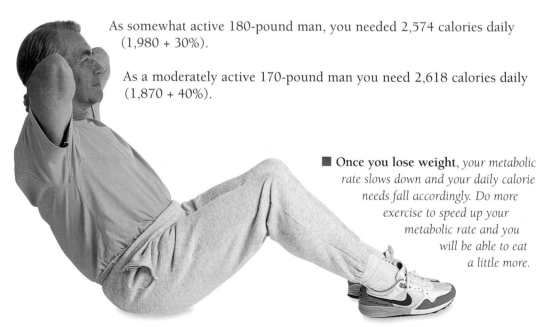

As somewhat active 180-pound man, you needed 2,574 calories daily (1,980 + 30%).

As a moderately active 170-pound man you need 2,618 calories daily (1,870 + 40%).

■ **Once you lose weight**, *your metabolic rate slows down and your daily calorie needs fall accordingly. Do more exercise to speed up your metabolic rate and you will be able to eat a little more.*

Look at your activity diary

If you kept an activity diary for a week or more, turn to that page now. How many calories did you expend in that week? Was it spread out evenly over all seven days or did you do most of your sweating on a single day or over the weekend? There's no wrong answer to my second question. It's simply an important piece of information as you apply what you know about yourself.

Is there time in each day – say an extra half hour – for a bit more activity? Or is your weekly schedule such that weekends are the best time for exercise? Is there a particular part of the day that is better suited to activity? Are you too rushed in the morning or too tired at night? Do you work when other people play and vice versa? Does the availability of other members of your family or friends influence when you are more or less likely to be active?

INTERNET

www.phys.com/c_tools/
calculators4/01home/
calculators.htm

You can "crunch your numbers" at this web site by choosing an activity and entering the number of minutes you plan to do it. Click the calculator to find out how many calories you'll burn.

Here's a modest proposal: See if you can add 100 calories worth of activity to each day or a total of 700 calories to your week. Write down some things you like to do and check out one of the many online activity calculators. How many minutes of each one adds up to 100 calories? If it seems like too much, write in as much time as you think you can spend and promise yourself that you'll revisit this question at a later date. If you can do more, be my guest!

INTERNET

www.phys.com/fitness/
burnmore

Short on ideas? Here you'll find a quiz with a few easy questions. In return for your answers, you'll get a personalized analysis, complete with suggestions for what you can do to be more active.

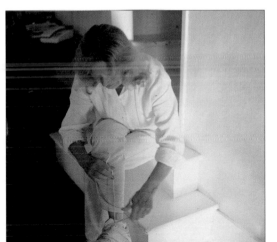

Now, divide your weekly total by 7 and subtract the answer from the number you circled as "My daily calorie goal." Circle the new number and label it "My daily calorie intake goal." That's the number you're going to work with when planning what you eat.

■ **One way to add** *an extra 700 calories' worth of activity to your week is to go for a brisk half-hour walk each day.*

Plan your daily calorie intake

THE NEXT STEP IS OBVIOUS. *Take out your food diary and compare your daily calorie intake goal with your actual daily calorie intake. The result may shock you.*

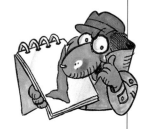

If your daily calorie intake fluctuated wildly over the course of a week, divide the weekly total by 7 to get a daily average.

Subtract the goal from the actual. That's how many calories you have to get off your plate. For example, suppose you averaged 4,000 calories a day, but your goal to lose the amount of weight you want in the time you want is 2,500 calories a day:

4,000 – 2,500 = 1,500

You need to eat 1,500 fewer calories each day.

Can you do it? If it seems like it will be just too hard, increase the number of days you'll do it in until you come up with a daily calorie goal that is feasible. Once you have a calorie goal that feels realistic, let's figure out how you can reach it most, if not all, days.

Keep it flexible

None of this is cast in stone. Remember, this is your first draft, subject to revision. And even after you have solidified your plan, you should allow yourself to make changes. If you are too rigid, you will regard a lapse or two as a total failure. That may lead you to give up entirely.

Set a short-term daily calorie goal and promise yourself to reassess it after 30 or 60 or 90 days.

You may want to slow the pace of your weight-loss or set a less ambitious long-term goal. In all likelihood, though, once you start eating and exercising more sensibly – and especially once you start losing weight – you will be in a different frame of mind. What seemed simply too challenging on day one may seem effortless on day 45.

Make some menus

When I was feeding a family of five, my biggest challenge was coming up with healthful and taste-tempting ideas day after day. Every once in a while I'd sit down with the family and ask them what they liked best to eat.

INTERNET

www.calorieking.com

Can't think of what to cook? Check out this web site for some healthy low-fat recipes.

We'd make a list of main meals, vegetables and other side dishes, desserts, and snacks. We'd post the list on the bulletin board and whenever ideas were in short supply, I'd pick one from column A and one from column B, etc. We made sure to include choices that ranged from quick and easy to major undertakings, economical to extravagant, and ingredients that were available in various seasons.

Do something similar for yourself, but instead of consulting your family, consult your calorie counter. Write down foods and food combinations you like.

1. Emphasize low-calorie, low-fat choices.

2. Think about lower-fat cooking methods, like steaming, boiling, poaching, rack grilling, and microwaving instead of frying, sautéing, and drowning food in sauces and gravies.

3. Use lower-fat alternatives.

4. Include snacks in your list, but make them low-cal.

Make a list of your personal food heroes and villains.

Food heroes are low-calorie, high-bulk foods in each of the food groups that you find delicious, tempting, satisfying, and easy to get your hands on. The villains are calorie-dense foods you can't stop eating once you start. Be sure your list includes lots of heroes. And banish as many of the villains as you think you can.

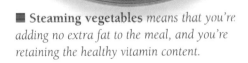

■ **Steaming vegetables** *means that you're adding no extra fat to the meal, and you're retaining the healthy vitamin content.*

Having detailed menus is good insurance against freelance bingeing. If you know what you're supposed to eat at any given meal, you can purchase the ingredients and prepare the right number and size of portions. Simply opening the refrigerator when you are hungry can be as dangerous as walking into a lion's den!

Prepackaged diet meals

The supermarket is full of diet meals with strictly metered portions. These can range from frozen entrées to snack bars and cans of diet shake. Many of the commercial diet plans have their own meal packages.

There is nothing wrong with using these, and for you, there may be a lot that is right. On the one hand, they may be more expensive than home-cooked meals. On the other, they are quick and easy to prepare and many of them are highly portable. Slipping a can or foil-wrapped bar into your backpack or attaché case may be the best insurance against a supersized burger and fries when you're on the run.

Some people don't find these foods particularly appetizing, but others may think they're delicious, or at least reasonably edible. And there's no question that toting up the calories is easier. Just read the label and jot down the info in your food diary. You may want to rely on them exclusively, occasionally, or not at all. It's really up to you.

Plan a day

Start out by planning a single day's eating. How many meals will you eat? The standard answer is three, but does that reflect your reality? Remember: Snacks are meals. Does the evidence in your food diary say you eat five or six or even more times each day? Can you cut out one or two of them?

Maybe more frequent, but smaller, meals is a good idea for you. If you often get hungry between meals, plan for that. It does not matter how often you eat as long as the total daily calories are within your goal. There is even some evidence that eating more often will help you lose weight, since revving up your digestion burns calories in the process.

■ **Breakfast** *is essential to start up the metabolism. Half a grapefruit, a bowl of sugar-free cereal with low-fat milk, and coffee is one way to start the day.*

THINK ABOUT SUBSTITUTES

For every food you like to eat, there is probably a lower-calorie alternative. In some cases, it may be a simple matter of eating less. In other cases, you can make an exchange that will satisfy your craving without putting you over your daily calorie goal. Here are a few alternatives. (Calories are average per serving.)

| Instead of | | Try | |
Food	Calories	Food	Calories
Large burger	560	Regular burger	270
Large fries	450	Small fries	210
Thick-crust pizza	350	Thin-crust pizza	220
Creamy French dressing	110	Oil and vinegar dressing	90
Deluxe ice cream	200	Low-fat ice cream	90
Chocolate shake	360	Low-fat chocolate milk	160
Cappuccino	70	Espresso	4
Fruit salad in heavy syrup	95	Cantaloupe	50
Peanuts	160	Pretzels	110
Baked potato w/ sour cream	270	Baked potato w/ nonfat yogurt	235
Chicken breast with skin	300	Chicken breast without skin	190
Fried egg	100	Poached egg	80
Chicken noodle soup	100	Chicken broth	30
Tuna with mayonnaise	160	Tuna with yogurt	70

Do not skip breakfast. This is a tempting strategy, but not a good one.

If you're like most people, breakfast is 8 or more hours after the last time you ate. Your body needs some fuel to get you started on your day. It doesn't have to be a huge meal, but it should feature some carbohydrates and something to drink, at the very least.

Begin a new food diary page, but instead of writing what you ate, write in what you plan to eat. Put in the time, the number of servings, and the calories. And then add up the calories. If the total is too high, decrease the servings or substitute another food. It's a good idea to use a pencil for this exercise, since you'll probably have to do a lot of revising.

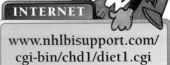

INTERNET

www.nhlbisupport.com/
cgi-bin/chd1/diet1.cgi

The National Heart, Lung, and Blood Institute has a handy "Create-a-Diet Activity" that will walk you through this process step by step.

Write it all down

THE BEST STRATEGY *for sticking to a plan is to keep a record. This may seem cumbersome and time-consuming, and I'll be the first to admit that it is.*

Your food and exercise diaries will be the most valuable tools in your weight-loss effort.

Writing down everything you eat and do in the way of exercise will:

a Help you see the truth in black-and-white

b Keep you honest, in case you "forget" something you ate or embellish something you did

c Motivate you

d Help you focus on where your problems lie

e Help you recognize triggers and unhealthy behavior patterns

f Help you analyze the effectiveness of your plan

g Try it for a while. Before long, your new, healthy habits will become ingrained.

h On the evening of the first day, after you've eaten your last bite, plan your eating and exercise for the rest of the week.

Trivia...

Did you know that exercise can be habit-forming? Physical exertion releases chemicals in the brain called endorphins. The specialized brain cells that attract them are the same that attract such powerful addictive drugs as opium and morphine. Endorphins are even more addictive than morphine, 200 times more so according to some experts. After a while your brain can become dependent on the exercise habit and beg you for more.

■ **Although it may** *seem time-consuming at first, tracking your calorie intake, and making revisions, in your food diary will really help your diet.*

244

A double-entry ledger

For the first week at least, your food and exercise diary should be like a double-entry ledger. There are sample food and activity pages in the back of this book that you can photocopy, or use as models for ones you make yourself. The first column is what you plan to eat or do; the second is what you actually ate or did. It's the best way to analyze what's working and what is not.

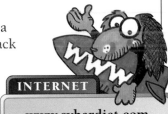

INTERNET

www.cyberdiet.com

You'll find calorie counts for more foods than you can eat at this web site.

If you possibly can, carry your food and activity diary pages with you. If this is not practical, use index cards and transfer the information into your weight loss notebook at the end of the day.

Write down everything that goes into your mouth and everything you do that qualifies as activity beyond what you usually do each day.

Daily food diary

Day **MONDAY** Date **9/11**

BREAKFAST Time *7.30am*

PLANNED	Calories	ACTUAL	Calories
coffee 1 cup	5	coffee 1 cup	5 cal
2 percent milk 1 oz	15	half & half 1 oz	40 cal
toast 2 slices	150	bagel (med) 3 oz	240 cal
jam 1 tbs	55	cream cheese 2 tbs	100 cal
orange juice 8 oz	110	orange juice 8 oz	110 cal
Total	335		495

COMMENTS

■ **Get used to keeping a** *double-entry ledger, putting down what you are aiming to eat in the left-hand column and what you actually consume in the right-hand column.*

Always keep track of your calorie intake. Use your calorie counter, or check one of the online counters. Don't cheat! Remember to count calories according to serving size. An overstuffed ham sandwich is not a serving; neither is a half carton of ice cream, nor an entire bunch of grapes. If you eat out, take advantage of the many calorie counters that list items sold at national chains. Keep track of how much water you're drinking and pour some more if you're not logging your daily minimum.

According to the medical experts, you can figure out how much water you need by dividing your weight in half to get the approximate number of fluid ounces you should drink.

So, if you weigh 140 pounds, that's 70 fluid ounces, or about 9 cups of water. Drink up!

Don't get discouraged if you fail to live up to your own expectations. Remember, this is a first draft. Learn from the differences between the two columns, and make notes in the comments column about what was going on. For example:

a) Did you wait until you were too hungry to eat sensibly?

b) Were you away from home or in a setting where food choice was limited?

c) Was there something stressful or otherwise triggering that caused you to violate your own rules?

d) Were you tempted by unsupportive companions?

e) Did you miss a planned exercise session because you were too busy or out of town?

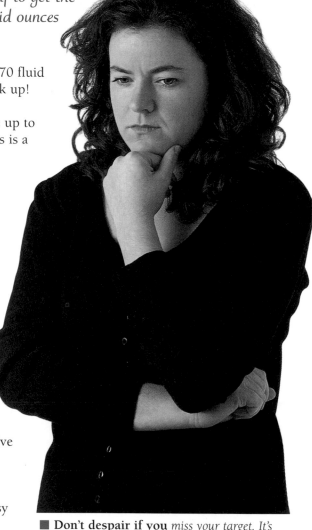

■ **Don't despair if you** *miss your target. It's important to keep yourself feeling positive and start each new day in an optimistic frame of mind.*

(f) Were you less active than usual because you were feeling ill?

(g) Did the weather sabotage your planned activity?

(h) Did you feel too sore because your previous exercise was too strenuous?

Think of the first week of your diet as a tryout.

If you lose some weight, that's great, but the main idea is to see how well you can live with what you've outlined for yourself. In the next part of this book, we'll be using what you learned to make a plan for the long term.

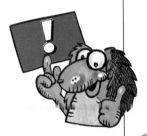

A simple summary

✔ The best weight-loss plan is one that is designed with you specifically in mind.

✔ BMR plus lifestyle percentage serves as a good ballpark figure for how many calories your body needs to consume each day to survive.

✔ In order for you to lose some weight, you first need to take in fewer calories than your body actually uses.

✔ Once you've set a weight-loss goal, spread that loss over a reasonable period of time.

✔ Plan some menus and sketch out an exercise plan for the first week.

✔ Keep a double-entry food and activity diary to help you evaluate your plan.

✔ Use the first week as a test to see if this is a plan you can live with.

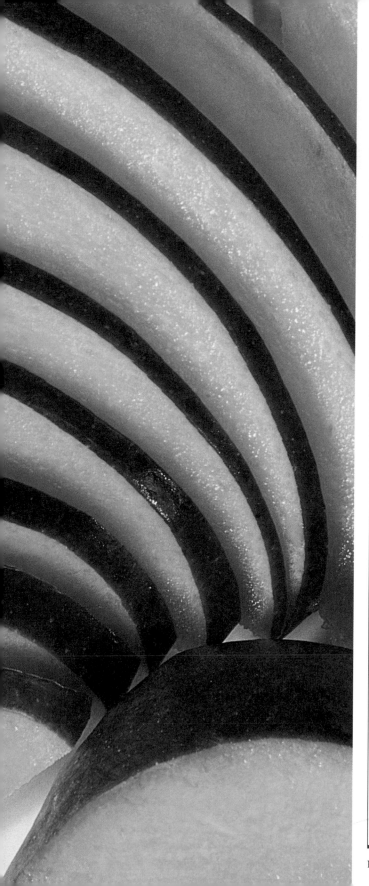

PART
FIVE

FRESH FRUIT: A HEALTHFUL SNACK IN MODERATION

DOING IT

YOU DIDN'T THINK I'd desert you as soon as you started your weight-loss campaign, did you? Living with a diet day-to-day is the hardest part about losing weight. Embarking on a plan to become fitter can be daunting. You need all the *encouragement* you can get.

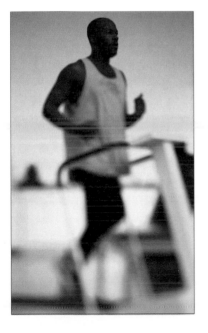

In this section, there's a pep talk focusing on *motivation* and *support*, two essentials for any effort. Find advice and encouragement on planning menus, monitoring your behavior and progress, and a section on turning your refrigerator into a diet ally instead of your worst enemy. Find ways to fit exercise into your busy life and *keep it interesting* and safe. Finally, learn what to do about lapses in your exercise schedule when they happen.

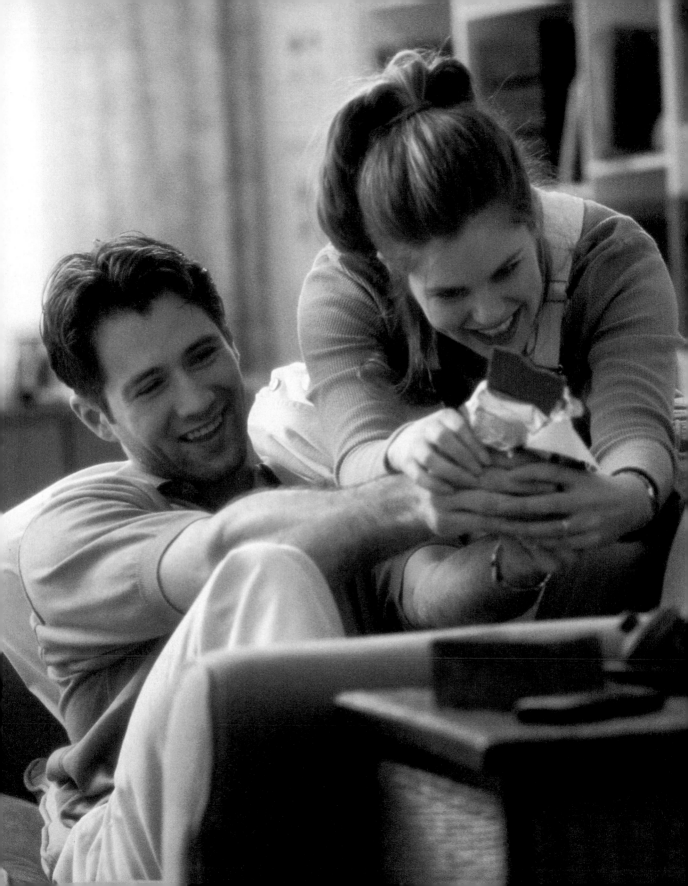

Chapter 15

Pep Talk

Y OU'RE FACING A BIG CHALLENGE NOW, and it's time to whip up your enthusiasm. There is no question that getting ready psychologically is an important key to weight-loss success. You know you should lose weight, you know how much you want to lose, and you know how you're going to go about doing it. All you need now is the will to win.

In this chapter...

✓ Motivate

✓ Evaluate

✓ Get support

✓ Give it time to work

✓ Monitor your progress

✓ On your mark, get set ...

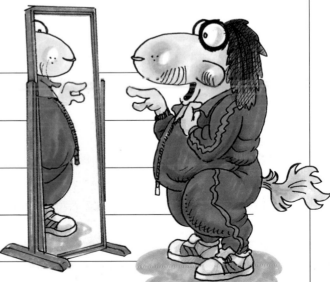

THE SUPPORT OF FAMILY AND FRIENDS CAN BE HELPFUL IN TIMES OF TEMPTATION

Motivate

THOMAS EDISON CALLED GENIUS *"one percent inspiration and 99 percent perspiration."* *When it comes to weight loss, I'd add motivation to that equation. I hope you'll be perspiring as well as eating more wisely, but what you'll need to keep going is to keep yourself motivated. The big question is "Why are you doing this?"*

Everyone has different reasons for wanting to lose weight. Knowing your personal reasons will help you keep your eyes on the prize.

Ask yourself why you want to lose weight. Are you doing it:

■ For your self-esteem?

■ For your health?

■ For your loved ones?

■ To improve your social life?

■ To improve your appearance?

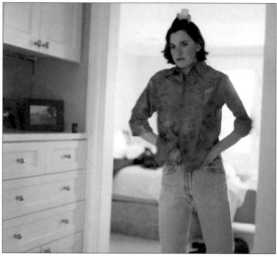

■ **Being able to fit back** *into a favorite old pair of jeans will bring a tremendous sense of achievement. As you pursue your weight-loss program, keep such goals in mind to really spur you on.*

You may want to lose weight for one or more of these reasons or for others I have not listed. Think about it and then take out your weight-loss notebook. On a new page, write down your reasons for wanting to weigh less than you do now.

Long-range and short-range motivators

The reasons I have listed fall into the category of long-range motivators. They are life changes that losing weight will help accomplish. If you are the sort of person who is inspired by long-range goals, this may be all you need.

Most of us, however, need to be reminded on a daily basis why we are working hard on a long project. That's where short-range motivators come in.

Try to break your reasons into small pieces. For example, if improving your self-esteem is an aim, a good place to start is by keeping a promise you make to yourself 3 days out of 7. If your health is an issue, a reasonable short-range goal would be exercising in your target heart rate zone twice a week.

Jot down as many motivators as you can think of, but be sure they are the ones that work for you. Think of your list of motivators as a work in progress. As you achieve some of your goals, you may want to add new ones. And the more success you have, the more motivated you will find you become.

Post your list of motivators on your mirror or somewhere else you're likely to see it often. Or slip them in your wallet or engagement calendar, or wherever else you will run across them when you could use a boost.

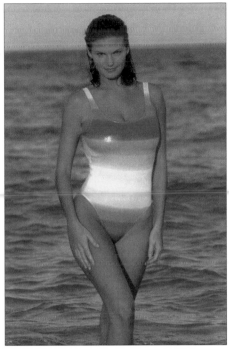

■ **Do everything you can** *to remind yourself why you are trying to lose weight. Cut out pictures of slender and fit-looking people and tack them up around the house.*

What about willpower?

Willpower is a buzzword often used when it comes to diet. Surely you've heard this one: "The most effective exercise is to push yourself away from the dinner table." The failure of willpower is often used as an insult to those who are overweight. The simple fact is that this negative label hurts more than it helps.

Many weight-loss experts reject the idea of willpower and doubt that it is a valid feature of human psychology.

Experts dispute that willpower is something some people "have" and others do not. Instead, they recommend strategies for changing behavior. These include:

a Keeping a food diary

b Eating purposefully and mindfully

c Being aware of the connection between moods and behaviors

d Distracting yourself from eating with other activities

Reward yourself

Virtue may be its own reward, but most of us like to have something a bit more tangible. So don't forget to reward yourself whenever you achieve one of your goals.

Rewards can be as simple and symbolic as a gold star or a smiley face in your notebook or calendar. They can be a special treat that has nothing to do with losing weight, like an evening out or a new book or CD. You could decide on something really big – a weekend getaway, perhaps – and put away a bit of money each time you achieve a short-range goal. Or give yourself a present that will add enjoyment to your new way of life. No, not a banana spilt when you lose a pound!

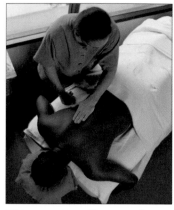

■ **Treat yourself** *to something you really enjoy, such as a pampering massage, when you achieve a weight-loss goal.*

Maybe you'd feel rewarded by buying an article of clothing you never thought you'd be able to wear. How about a new workout outfit? A pair of shiny spandex leggings or a biceps-revealing tank top might be just the ticket. If you're not ready for a new look, how about a massage or a facial? You know best what turns you on and what feels like a treat. Make a list of some small and big rewards you can look forward to when you've passed a weight-loss milestone.

Evaluate

WITHOUT A PLAN, motivation is little more than pie in the sky. That pie might not pack as many calories as the deep-dish apple kind, but it won't help you lose weight either. You need to match your aims to your abilities.

Making changes

Losing weight in a healthy and sensible way means making big changes in your daily habits. It requires a new attitude toward eating and exercise. A survey conducted by the Calorie Control Council covered the reasons why people fail to achieve and maintain their desired weight.

In a Calorie Control Council survey, more than half the people who responded said they couldn't obtain their desired weight because of lack of exercise.

Many of the reasons had to do with food and eating behavior:

- Snacking too much

- Eating too many high-fat foods

- Bingeing

- Overeating at mealtimes

- Eating for emotional reasons

- Having trouble eating properly at restaurants

- Reducing fat, but not calories

- Reducing calories, but not fat

Does one or more of these reasons apply to you? Will making changes in these areas get you in the weight-loss frame of mind? Start a new page in your weight-loss notebook. Write "Changes" across the top and divide the page into two columns. Call one column "Small Changes" and the other "Big Changes."

Make a list of things you know you have to do differently. *Be specific.* "Eat less" is a change, but not one you can measure. Same with "Exercise more." Attach some numbers to those concepts and you'll give yourself a yardstick to measure by. Be positive. That is, go heavy on the "do's" and light on the "don'ts."

Your list of small changes might include:

- Drink eight to ten glasses of water a day

- Get off the bus one stop earlier and walk the rest of the way home every other day

- Make menus for every day

- Limit restaurant meals to once a week

- Snack on pretzels instead of chips

- Eliminate 50 calories from each meal every day

- Ride bike for a half hour on the weekend.

Your list of big changes might include:

- The kitchen closes at 9 p.m.

- Join a gym

- Save french fries for special occasions: one serving no more than once a month

- Eat one serving only of every food

- Eat only from my menu—no unplanned noshing

- Eliminate 2,000 calories from each week

- Learn salsa dancing

These are just a few suggestions. Some of my small changes may feel like big changes to you, and vice versa. Or the things you need to change may be very different. So make your own list by thinking about the places that food and activity occupy in your life. Use your sample food and exercise diaries to see where some of the problems lie and where there is room for improvement.

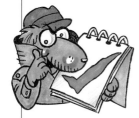

The small changes to your daily routine should be things you know you can do; all that's required is that you make a list. The big changes are more challenging. There may be practical and psychological barriers to surmount, and you may have to try more than once before you succeed.

You may find it helpful to put the big changes in some sort of order – from easiest to most difficult, from least to most important to you, from the ones you want to try first to those you'll put off for a while.

This is a stick-up

Buy a pack of index cards or a pad of stick-up notes and write one of the changes on each. You might find it helpful to write the change on one side and keep a record of your progress toward this change on the other. Post the cards or stick-up notes on a bulletin board, a mirror, or the door of your refrigerator – anywhere you are likely to see them. You might even want to put some inside your refrigerator or stick one or two on particularly dangerous foods. There's nothing like finding some serious reading matter on a box of chocolates to give you pause!

Another idea that might work better for you is to write your changes on a calendar. It can be a wall calendar or one you carry with you. Each time you make one of these changes, check it off or stick a gold star on it!

Give yourself some choices

Experts call making changes "behavior modification," and they believe it is the key to permanent weight loss and improved fitness. They also know that you can't "just say no," and expect it to work all the time or even most of the time.

The best thing to do is give yourself alternatives.

If you spend your evenings watching television, think about some more active things you can do instead. If your favorite leisure-time activity is watching sports, how about becoming a player rather than a spectator, at least some of the time? If you get together with friends for coffee and donuts, how about meeting for an hour of dancing instead? If you lie on the beach with a book, why not join the beach volleyball game or toss a Frisbee™ with your friends? If your normal bedtime snack is milk and cookies, allow yourself an apple and say goodnight.

Make a list of eating and leisure-time behaviors you regularly engage in. Circle the ones that are positive and cross out the ones that are not. Replace those you've crossed out with satisfying alternatives. Make yourself some cards or stick-up notes that read "Instead of (bad habit), try (good habit)" and post them around the house or office.

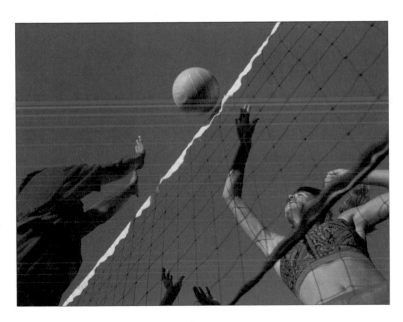

■ **Volleyball is** *a vigorous, fun sport. It uses the whole body, so gives all your muscles, including your heart, a good workout.*

Your hopes and fears

Back in Chapter 7 when you were exploring what food means to you, you wrote about your hopes and fears about losing weight. Now that you are closer to doing that, you may want to reread and reevaluate what you wrote. Have your hopes become more realistic or more ambitious? Are your fears diminished or have you added new ones?

Try to turn each hope and fear into a positive, motivating statement. For example, if you wrote that you are afraid that losing weight will be too difficult, write something like "Losing weight may be difficult, but I am ready to face the challenge." If you wrote that being slimmer will mean you can wear a bathing suit without embarrassment, write something like "Bathing suit season is just 10 weeks away, and I'll be ready for it."

Write each of these positive statements on an index card and post them in prominent places in your home or office. Or make each one of them a motto of the day and write it on your calendar.

Get support

NOW'S THE TIME to gather the members of your team. Check the "Friends of My Diet" list you made in Chapter 1 and tell them that you are beginning your weight-loss plan. Ask them to give you as much encouragement as they can in the days ahead. You may want to let them know the details of your plan and tell them what they can do to help.

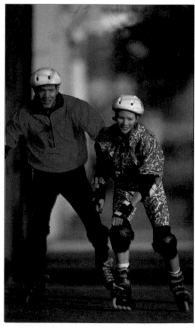

■ If you'd like them to hold off on food-based gatherings, tell them

■ If you have special food requests when they are preparing meals, give them a list

■ If you want a witness at your weigh-ins, arrange a time and place

■ If you want someone to take your measurements, hand over the tape measure

■ **Get a friend** *to go inline skating with you, if it's a sport that appeals. But be sure to wear protective gear.*

- If you want company while you walk, run, bike, or dance, make a date

- If you want them to ask you how you're doing, let them know

- If you want to make time for exercise, ask them to take over some of your tasks or responsibilities

Look into an online chat. You may wish to "lurk" for the first few days, but when you have the courage, take the plunge and join in the discussion. Virtual diet buddies can be as helpful as people you see every day, and maybe even more so

INTERNET

boards.excite.com

Excite is one of many web portals that host online message boards. Click on "Health" and then "Diet and Nutrition" or "Exercise and Fitness" to find people just like you who need and want to give support.

Do not let anyone discourage you from your weight-loss plans.

If you have friends or family who are skeptical of your plan or who seem to enjoy undermining your efforts, don't share your hopes and plans with them. Let them be surprised by the change they will surely notice in the future. Remember the words of my aerobics instructor: "Stay away from negative people. You know who they are."

Give it time to work

ONCE YOU GET STARTED, *try to balance determination with patience. That's the best way to get over the rough spots.*

Most likely, you will quickly shed a few pounds, maybe even in the first week.

Much of this will be water, as your body adjusts to your new way of eating. Still, a good portion will be true weight loss, as your body draws on stored fat to make up for the fact that you're taking in fewer calories than you need to function. You may not see a difference for a while, but the scale will tell the story.

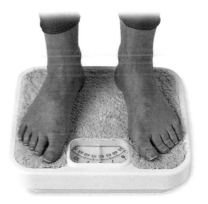

■ **As your clothes** *start to feel looser you'll know that you're losing weight. The scale will confirm it.*

It usually takes time for your shape to catch up to your weight loss. You may begin to notice that your clothes are a bit looser or someone may ask if you've lost weight because your face seems thinner. But don't expect to notice any of these changes in the first week or two.

The flip side of the coin

The good news about this rapid initial weight loss is that it will cheer you on, providing some instant motivation. The bad news is that it won't last for long. In a short while, your metabolism will gear down to compensate for the lower calorie intake. The rate of your weight loss will slow and eventually stop, unless you "fool" your body by increasing your level of activity.

How quickly people arrive at a weight-loss plateau varies. Typically, it comes after about 10 pounds are lost, though the more you have to lose, the longer it will take before you hit a plateau.

The important thing is not to get discouraged.

Stick to your plan and be patient. Remember you are making big changes meant to last a lifetime. The main task of the first few weeks of your weight-loss plan is to learn how to live with it, to figure out what works and what does not, and to observe how well you are able to meet the commitment you have made. If you find yourself getting discouraged, call on your pep squad. Talk to a friend, seek out advice, or vent your frustration in an online chat or in-person support group.

Expect lapses

No matter how motivated you are, no matter how determined you are, you may sometimes do something you know you shouldn't, or fail to do what you have planned. You might miss an exercise session or help yourself to seconds out of habit rather than hunger. You might give in to a temptation or say "yes" when you should have said "no." You are, after all, only human.

The worst thing you can do is treat a lapse as a failure and give up your weight-loss plan entirely. Instead, treat it as a minor transgression. Try to make up for it by eating less at the next meal or the next day, exercising harder or longer at the next session, or readjusting one of your short-term goals.

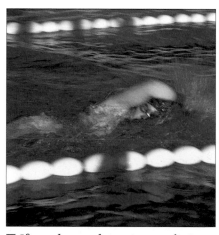

■ **If you have a lapse** *in your dieting, don't give up, just dedicate more time to exercising. Doing a few more laps in the pool will make all the difference.*

Above all, forgive yourself and keep going. If you can learn something from the lapse, all the better. Maybe an after-work exercise session isn't right for you. Would it be better to get your activity in at lunchtime or in the morning? Maybe working out every day is too ambitious right now. Maybe having lunch with your coworkers every day is just too tempting. Maybe there are too many snack foods in your cupboard and it's time to clear them out.

Remember that an explanation is not an excuse.

It's a good idea to try to understand what went wrong. It's a good idea to forgive yourself. But it is not a good idea to blame the lapse on outside factors and do nothing to avoid it in future.

Monitor your progress

KEEPING A WEIGHT-LOSS JOURNAL *is the simplest and most effective way to stay on track. A daily food and activity diary is a must. Periodically updating your personal database is also a good idea.*

Continue to use your weight-loss notebook for your daily diaries or do it on index cards or make photocopies of the journal blanks in the back of this book. If you prefer, you can make up your own forms. Whatever you do, make sure your diary is portable, easy to use, and suited to your own plan.

INTERNET

www.nhlbi.nih.gov/ health/public/heart

The National Heart, Lung, and Blood Institute has a food and activity diary blank that you can print out in HTML or PDF versions. It shows a week at a glance, with space for breakfast, lunch, and dinner, activity, diet and activity goals, and comments about behavior.

Choose your time frame

When it comes to your personal database, you can decide whether to track your progress week-by-week or month-by-month.

Don't track your progress day-by-day.

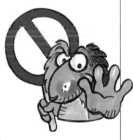

Weighing and measuring yourself every day will not give you the boost you need. Your weight can fluctuate by a pound or more on a daily basis. Significant and realistic loss will begin showing up from week to week, and will probably be most dramatic from month to month.

261

Weigh yourself on the first day of your weight-loss campaign and write the date. If you want, take your measurements and date those too. Other baseline figures should include your

■ **BMI**

■ **RHR** (resting heart rate)

■ **MHR** (maximum heart rate)

■ **THR** (target heart rate)

If you don't remember how to figure these out, look back at Chapter 8.

Allow space for updates, weekly or monthly, as you choose. Every time you take a new measurement, date it. You might also want to buy some highlighters and designate one color for improvement, one for no change, and a third for movement in the opposite direction. Ideally, you'll see nothing but improvement, but you will in any event be able to tell at a glance how your campaign is going.

Commentary

Make space for comments, either on your daily diary or on a separate page in your notebook. Jot down what works and what does not, moods that explain (but don't excuse) lapses, triggers that cause you to break your rules, things that will help you follow them.

It's a good idea to reevaluate your plan from time to time. Your comments and your colorful personal database will help you decide if revision is needed, and if so, what to revise.

After you've lived with your weight-loss plan for a month, you may want to reset your milestones. Maybe the weight is coming off faster than you expected. Maybe your improved fitness level makes it possible for you to exercise more vigorously. Or maybe you were unrealistic in your goals. The only way to know for sure is to do it.

On your mark, get set ...

NOW'S THE TIME. *Are you ready? Choose whatever it takes to get you started.*

■ Make it a New Year's resolution.

■ Give yourself a birthday, anniversary, or graduation present.

■ Begin it with the new day, week, month, or season.

But remember, there's no time like the present. If you find yourself putting off your weight-loss plan, ask yourself why it's always tomorrow and tomorrow and tomorrow.

Take out the contract you made back in Chapter 9 and reread it. Do you want to make any changes? If so, the time is now. Then sign it and date it, and get a witness.

Go!

A simple summary

✔ Motivation is the key to sticking to a weight-loss plan.

✔ Keep your motivation high by setting both short- and long-range goals.

✔ Focus on ways to modify your behavior as you replace bad habits with good ones.

✔ Reward yourself when you succeed; forgive yourself when you lapse.

✔ Get support from friends and family, or from your designated diet buddies.

✔ Give your plan enough time to work and do not allow a momentary lapse to throw you off course: Persistence and patience are just as important as motivation itself.

✔ Monitor your progress thoroughly. Nothing succeeds like success.

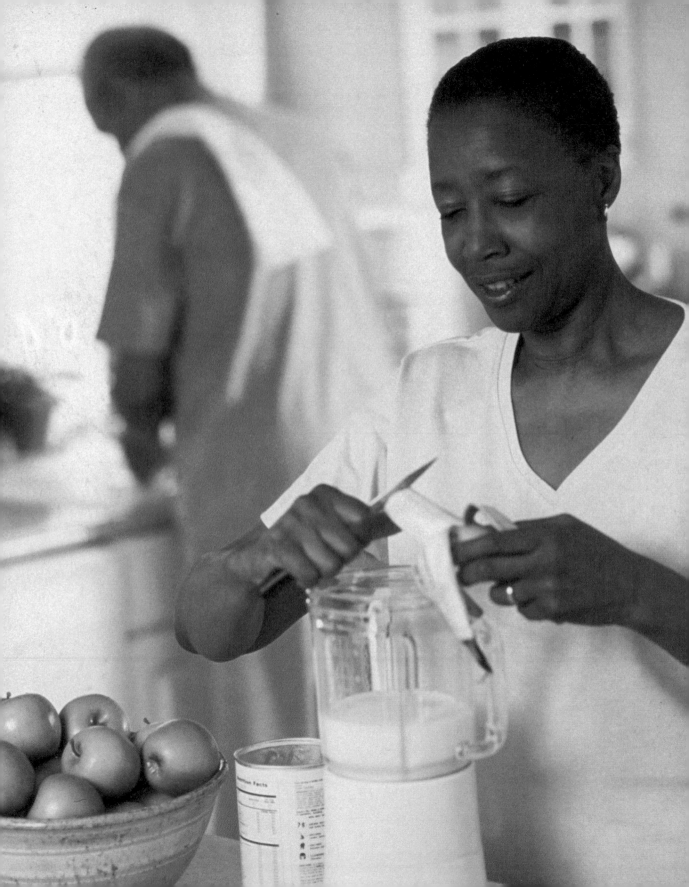

Chapter 16

Living With Your Diet

THINK OF THIS as "the first day of the rest of your life." This is the beginning of a new relationship with food and eating. The purpose of all the learning, thinking, and planning that went before is to help you change. Your new way of eating should be something you can live with. In this chapter, we'll look at a variety of ways you can make your diet fit into your life, or small and large changes you may have to make to fit your life to your diet.

In this chapter...

✓ Keeping your diary

✓ Planning meals

✓ Dealing with hunger

✓ Dealing with cravings

✓ At the supermarket

✓ You and your refrigerator

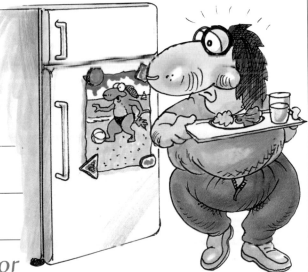

Keeping your diary

NOW IS NOT THE TIME to abandon your food diary. Instead, this is when it really comes into its own. Use it to record everything you eat and drink, including water. At least once a day, total up the calories you've taken in.

Keep comparing your intake with the goals you set for yourself. If you exceed them one day, try to correct that by eating less the next. If you find yourself repeatedly overeating, take a hard look at why. Have you set your sights too high? Are you making poor food choices? Are you in places and with people that do not support your weight-loss efforts? In short, do you need to revise your plan or develop strategies to make it easier to follow?

Mindfulness

Snacking, eating on the run, tasting while you cook and prepare food, eating while reading or watching television are all habits that disconnect your mind from your mouth. Overeating is often a matter of being unaware, or ignoring, how much you are packing in. Making menus, planning meals, keeping a food diary, and many of the other seemingly time-consuming behaviors I recommend are all ways to become more mindful about your eating habits. This means being aware of what you do. And making conscious decisions about whether to do it.

■ **Menu planning** is an excellent strategy for giving you control over what you eat, since you can check the calories in the ingredients in advance.

Before you reject these strategies as "just too much trouble," think of them as weight-loss aids. Give them a try. I am certain you will find the time you spend pays off not only in pounds but in perception. These strategies are important parts of the behavior modification that is essential to make your weight loss a permanent gain.

Think slim, think fit, then think again before entering!

FRIDGE NOTE

INTERNET

onhealth.webmd.com

If you'd like help keeping your diary, there's an interactive Diet and Fitness Journal at this web site.

Planning meals

IN THE LAST CHAPTER *I urged you to make menus ahead of time for every meal you plan to eat and to eat nothing you have not planned. That strategy will eliminate what is for most of us the major pitfall in achieving and maintaining a healthy weight. I call it freelance noshing. What it amounts to is letting your calorie intake get out of control.*

It is of course possible to plan meals down to the last dollop of mayonnaise and still eat far more than you should.

The secret of success is to apply healthy diet principles to your meal planning and to count the calories in everything you plan to eat.

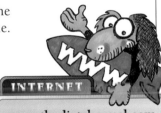

■ **When planning meals** *in advance, make sure each day's menu is different so you don't get bored.*

But don't give up meal planning and calorie counting just yet, even if they sound time-consuming and tedious. Do it a day or a week at a time. You may not do a perfect job, but as you see the payoff in more rational eating and the beginnings of your weight loss, you will have the motivation to continue.

In time, you may be able to relax the routine, but only if you adopt the good habits that go along with the job. You will begin to know approximately how many calories are in the things you regularly eat. You will develop a repertoire of dishes and full meals that you prepare time and again. And you will abandon many of the reckless eating behaviors that made you overweight in the first place.

Menu building

An easy way to begin is to develop some menu modules – meal components that you can mix and match for variety. Look in cookbooks for low-fat ideas and recipes, and use your calorie counter. Set aside an hour or so to do this. It'll be time well spent. Keep your calorie-counting book on hand, or dial up an online version.

INTERNET

www.thedietchannel.com

You may find yourself turning on The Diet Channel throughout your weight-loss campaign. It is full of valuable information. Click on "The Best Diet Analysis Tools on the Web" to find calorie needs calculators and much more.

In a new page of your weight-loss notebook, list all the categories of foods you can think of. For example:

- Beverages
- Snacks
- Breakfast foods
- Salads
- Soups
- Vegetable side dishes

- Grains and starches
- Pasta dishes
- Meats
- Desserts
- Sandwiches
- Quick meals

Under each heading, write all the foods you like to eat. Next, find the per-serving calorie count for each food and write it in. It's also a good idea to indicate what a serving amounts to – how many pieces or ounces or cups or tablespoons. Leave space in each category to make additions as you broaden your food choices.

But first, cross out those foods whose calorie counts are too high. These you'll have to say no to, at least for now.

USING LOW-CAL COOKING METHODS

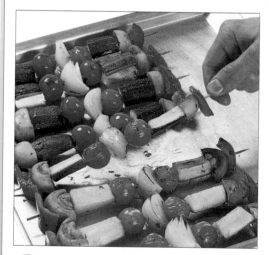

 Try not to fry

Bake or grill food to minimize the fat content. To help preserve vitamins, cook fruit and vegetables in their skins.

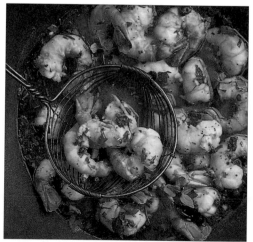

 Cook without fats

Use stock and wine, citrus juice, or aromatic sauces to replace oil when quick cooking foods for flavor minus the fat.

If you find yourself crossing out foods you can't live without, try to make them more acceptable.

(a) Will you be satisfied with a half or even smaller portion?

(b) Is there a lower-calorie version that tastes almost as good?

(c) Can you use a different cooking method to reduce the calorie burden?

(d) Can you substitute some of the high-calorie ingredients?

(e) Can you use the dish as a special occasion treat?

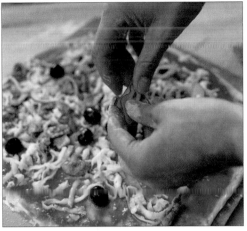

■ **If you can't face** *life without pizza, why not buy some dough bases and top them at home? Choose your toppings sensibly and you'll be able to enjoy pizza without packing in the calories.*

Apply healthy diet principles

You may want to review the basics of nutrition in Chapter 4 and the healthy diet principles in Chapter 11. Take an especially good look at the food pyramid, which is a wonderful model for menu planning. Ask yourself:

(a) Do your categories include foods from each of the food pyramid groups?

(b) Are there enough selections that contain complex carbohydrates?

(c) Do your choices de-emphasize fats and sugars, which should be eaten only sparingly?

(d) Are there enough fruits and vegetables on your list to provide variety along with the suggested number of servings? If not, add some more.

(e) Have you chosen cooking methods that will reduce the fat in what you prepare?

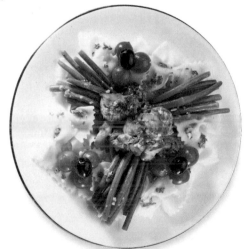

■ **Fresh grilled tuna** *with pasta and vegetables is a meal that's low in fat yet provides a good balance of carbohydrates, protein, fiber, vitamins, and minerals.*

WHAT IS A SERVING ANYWAY?

The USDA has a very clear definition of what a serving is. All the recommendations on the food pyramid are based on this. So are the calorie counts on food packaging and in most calorie counters. If your definition of a serving is different, it's time to face the facts. Here's a sampling of what the USDA considers to be a serving of various foods by category:

Breads and cereals

- 1 slice of bread
- ½ English muffin
- 4 small crackers
- 1 ounce ready-to-eat cereal
- ½ cup cooked cereal, rice, or pasta

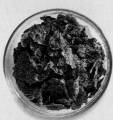

BRAN FLAKES

Vegetables

- ½ cup cooked vegetables
- ½ cup raw chopped vegetables
- 1 cup raw leafy vegetables
- ½–¾ cup vegetable juice

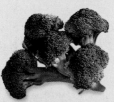

BROCCOLI

Fruits

- 1 medium fresh fruit (about 1 cup)
- ½ cup canned fruit
- ¼ cup dried fruit
- ½–¾ cup fruit juice

DRIED APRICOTS

Meat, fish, etc.

- 2–3 ounces cooked lean meat, poultry, or fish
- 2 eggs
- 7 ounces tofu
- 1 cup cooked legumes (dried beans, peas)
- 4 tablespoons peanut butter
- ½ cup nuts or seeds

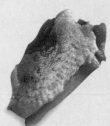

CHICKEN

Milk and dairy products

- 1 cup milk or yogurt
- 1 ounce cheese
- ½ cup cottage cheese
- ½ cup ice cream or frozen yogurt

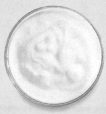

YOGURT

Learn to recognize a serving

If freelance noshing is the major pitfall of a healthful diet, portion overload runs a close second. A portion or serving is the amount of any food that a person would normally eat at a single sitting. Calorie counts are based on that serving size. A plate filled with a half-pound slab of beef and a huge mound of mashed potatoes is literally enough to feed a crowd, or at least two or three people.

Educate yourself about portion sizes of everything you eat. You can get this information from food packages, any calorie counter, and from the U.S. Department of Agriculture.

You won't always have access to a label, so it's a good idea to familiarize yourself with what a serving looks like on your plate. This will be especially important when you eat out, either in a restaurant or at another person's house, when you have less control over how much is served. The best way to do this is to dedicate some time in the kitchen, weighing and measuring out your favorite foods. Once again, your calorie counter is a vital reference.

If you don't already have one, buy a kitchen scale. Sets of graduated measuring cups and measuring spoons are essential too.

Begin by filling a plate with what you think is a serving of meat, vegetables, and a starch. Then weigh or measure each one, as appropriate, to see how close you come to the "correct" definition of a serving (see opposite page). You may be surprised.

KITCHEN SCALE

If you've overestimated serving sizes, weigh or measure out the correct amount and rearrange the plate. Look at it. Commit that picture to memory. Next, measure out one tablespoon of butter and put it on a plate. Do the same with one tablespoon of jam or jelly. You could even spread these on a slice of bread and see how far a tablespoon goes. Is this about how much you usually use? More? Less?

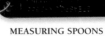

MEASURING SPOONS

Measure out a cup of yogurt. A half-cup of ice cream. Put each in a bowl and look at them. (Now put the ice cream back in the freezer or find someone else to eat it.)

271

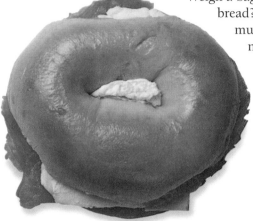

Weigh a bagel. How much more does it weigh than a slice of bread? Two times as much? Three? More? If you're a muffin eater, weigh one of the giants you have with mid-morning coffee and see how it compares to the one in your calorie counter. Is it twice as heavy? Then double the calories.

Cut a 1-ounce chunk or slice of cheese. Pour an ounce of your favorite breakfast cereal into a bowl. You get the idea. Do this as often as you have to with all the foods you typically eat.

Once you know how to recognize a serving on your plate or in your hand, you'll be better able to know how much you are really eating.

■ **Bagels are** *high in calories, so you might consider eating half a bagel or less.*

Portion-control patrol

Restaurants usually control portions by filling plates in the kitchen, although how full a plate is can range from minimal to heaping. In many homes, the usual custom is to set out large serving pieces containing more food than will – or should – be eaten at that meal, and to fill plates from there.

A simple way to exercise portion control is to fill your plate in the kitchen and then carry it into a different room to eat it.

Filling plates in the kitchen serves two purposes:

1. You can use a scale, measuring cups, and measuring spoons to monitor portion size. You may want to do this all the time or just for a while until you learn to recognize a serving on your plate.

2. It keeps extra food out of sight and out of reach. If you want more, you have to actually get up and walk back into the kitchen and deliberately serve yourself. That gives you time to think: "Am I really still hungry? Do I really want more lasagna?" In most cases, the answer is "No."

The answer to seconds should be NO!

If you have planned your menus based on single servings and allowed yourself that number of calories, second helpings amount to a second meal. And that's a meal you can't afford.

Soup and other filling starters

When planning meals, think about the sequence of what you eat. Remember the concept of calorie density we discussed back in Chapter 11? If you begin with filling but low-calorie foods – that is, foods that are less calorie dense – you will be satisfied with smaller amounts of foods that are more calorie dense.

Soups and salads are excellent first courses. The liquid in the soup and the bulkiness of the lettuce and other salad vegetables will make you feel full before you get to the main course. Drinking a glass of water or other low-cal beverage is another good idea.

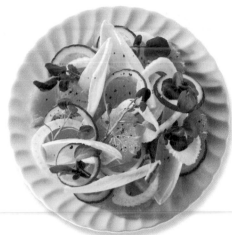

■ **Salads are ideal** *first courses. Make them interesting by mixing different flavors and textures.*

Mealtimes

Schedule your mealtimes and stick to that schedule. Don't forget to schedule your snacks. This is the best way to prevent freelance noshing. You definitely want to get out of the habit of eating when you are not hungry, but waiting too long for hunger to develop holds its own dangers. Feeling like you are "starving" too often leads to wolfing down your food. The result is that you eat far more than you intend and don't even notice that your hunger has passed.

The best time to eat is when you are hungry but not ravenous.

You may not be able to exercise total control over mealtimes. The needs of others in your household and requirements of your work may dictate when you eat. Do it as well as you can. Look at the food diary you kept for a week before beginning your diet. Are there any clues about times of day when you felt most hungry? Were there times when you were too hungry and ate irresponsibly as a result?

How many meals a day?

The traditional number is three, but most of us actually eat more than that. Remember, a snack is a meal. You can try to impose a three-a-day schedule, but don't assume this is the best way to go. There is evidence that more frequent but smaller meals are an aid to weight loss. Not only do you get the digestion benefit – it takes calories to burn calories – but you also stave off ravenous hunger and develop the habit of eating less at each sitting.

Whatever you do, don't skip breakfast. I've said this before, but it bears repeating. It's tempting to "save" some calories by eliminating this meal. Don't.

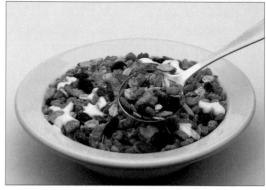

Your mother was right: Breakfast is the most important meal of the day. Unless you're a midnight snacker, morning finds you at the end of the longest between-meals stretch. The calories you consume at breakfast will save you from overdoing it later in the day.

■ **However busy you are**, *make time to eat breakfast. Your body needs an energy boost to get your metabolism in gear.*

Breakfast doesn't have to be huge and it doesn't have to take a lot of time. You can have a diet shake, poured from a can or one you blend yourself with yogurt, banana, a tablespoon of wheat germ, and an ounce or two of fruit juice. Or it can be a slice of whole-grain toast with a swipe of jam and a piece of fruit. Add a cup of coffee or tea, if that's what you like, or have a glass of water. It's your best insurance against "needing" a megamuffin by mid-morning.

Dealing with hunger

HUNGER IS THE BOGEYMAN that lurks in every dieter's background. Or, I should say, fear of hunger. When you eat, and especially when you eat unwisely, are you really hungry? Or are you eating because you're afraid you'll get hungry if you don't? Are you responding to physiological hunger or to an emotional hunger or other trigger?

Try to get into the habit of evaluating the hunger messages your brain sends out. How long has it been since you last ate? Did you eat breakfast? What else is going on right now? Are you bored, tense, anxious? Before you answer your hunger, take out your weight-loss notebook and write about it. Note the time, mood, and circumstances, and anything else that will give you insight. This is another act of mindfulness designed to help you deal with the challenge.

While you are eating

Physical fullness and mental satiety are not necessarily the same thing. Remember, it takes about 20 minutes for your brain to process and send the message that you are no longer hungry. You can shovel in a lot of food during that time if you're not careful.

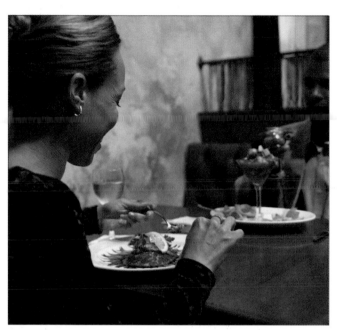

This is one of the best reasons to eat slowly. If you finish your meal before the 20 minutes elapse, you'll leave the table a lot fuller than necessary.

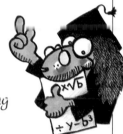

Your stomach can hold about 6 cups of food at a time. When you feel "full," you're probably nearing that capacity.

Listen to your body. Are you satisfied enough to stop eating? Do you want to continue because you are still hungry or because you're on a roller coaster and don't know how to stop it? Do you want more of the taste or more of the food? If it's mostly the taste you're after, take small bites and savor each morsel.

■ **It's a paradox**, *but one of the hardest times to deal with hunger is when you are eating. You may be hungry when you begin to eat, but do you know when the hunger stops? Can you stop eating then?*

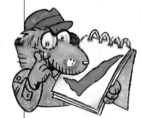

Eating slowly – pausing between mouthfuls and courses – is an effective strategy for dealing with hunger. It helps you tune into the subtleties of satiety.

Reschedule mealtimes

If you can be certain that what you're feeling is "real" hunger, you may want to consider changing when you eat. If a half hour will make the difference between simply being hungry and being hungry enough to eat a horse, plan meals a half hour earlier. If you can't seem to make it to the next meal without freelance noshing, schedule a series of small meals instead of three big ones.

TV DINNERS

It's as American as apple pie and just about as fattening. Eating while watching television is a habit worth breaking. I know this is a radical proposal, but I urge you to ban food from the television area.

The simple fact is that you cannot pay attention to the screen and to what you're eating at the same time. You would be amazed – and I hope appalled – by how many calories you can put away during a half-hour sitcom. If you don't believe me, monitor your eating and screen time for a week.

Kicking the habit won't be easy, I know. You'll be swimming against a tsunami of food and soft-drink commercials, cooking shows, and sports events (which have spawned a snack industry all their own). Not to mention the six o'clock news. Try to break the habit a day at a time, and ask your friends and family to help.

Make sure any eating you do is deliberate. Schedule, plan it, and eat what and when you intend to.

Keep track of everything that goes into your mouth and tote up the calories at the end of the day. Compare the total to your daily goal. If nothing else works, have a little something, but do it mindfully. Choose a food that will take the "edge" off your hunger. Look at the number of calories you've consumed so far that day and how many you have left before you reach your limit. Decide how much you can afford to borrow from later in the day. Measure out the amount, put it on a plate, and give all of your intention to eating it. Munching while you're doing something else is a way of denying that you're eating.

And when you're done, write down the calories you consumed. To keep yourself honest, you should subtract those calories from another meal that day so your daily total is unchanged. It's a little like borrowing from Peter to pay Paul.

■ **If you must eat something,** *choose a food that will take the edge off your hunger. Melon makes a good, refreshing choice.*

Dealing with cravings

DON'T MISTAKE HUNGER FOR A CRAVING. *Hunger is, or should be, a physiological response: Your body needs fuel. A craving is a psychological response: You feel like something sweet or crunchy or gooey or . . . whatever. Visions of devil's food cake swim in your head. You're thinking about salted peanuts or a nice juicy steak. Stop! Distract yourself. Do something else. Try one of these anti-craving strategies.*

(a) Pull out your food blacklist: If the food you crave is on it, remind yourself that you simply cannot eat this.

(b) Substitute: Try to find something that will satisfy the sensation without packing the same calorie load. Potato chips are crunchy, but so are thin slices of raw carrot. Chocolate is sweet, but so are strawberries. And if it must be chocolate, how about chocolate low-fat yogurt or chocolate skim milk?

■ **Chocolate is sweet,** *but eating strawberries is a much better way of overcoming a craving.*

(c) Distract yourself: If you can't get a craving out of your mind, take your mind somewhere else. Go for a walk, call a friend, pick up a book or magazine, get back to work, put on some music and dance.

(d) Try a delaying tactic: Cravings are usually a passing fancy, so it's worth trying to wait them out. See if you can put it off for 5 minutes. If you get through that, try another 5. The chances are good that the intensity of your craving will have subsided. If you can make it through 20 minutes, you're probably home free, since cravings tend to evaporate after that amount of time. That's one sure way to tell the difference between a craving and true hunger.

(e) Get support: Talk to one of your diet friends. Say you are in the throes of a craving and need some help.

■ **Phone a friend** *for encouragement when you're having a craving crisis. A little moral support can do wonders to help you get through a difficult time.*

277

f Save it as a reward: Say no now, and promise yourself you can have it when you have reached one of your milestones. If you can get through the week without giving in to your craving, make a date with it for Saturday night. And be sure to dress it up for the occasion. That means not eating it out of the bag or box. Take out your nicest plate or bowl, arrange the table in an attractive manner. And then sit down and eat this very special treat.

g Have just one bite: If all else fails, and it's eat it now or go off your diet, you may as well give in. Give in, but don't go crazy. Have a bit, a small bite. Taste it. Savor it. Then ask yourself, was that as good as I dreamed? Is that enough for now? Chances are the answers will be "No" and "Yes," in that order.

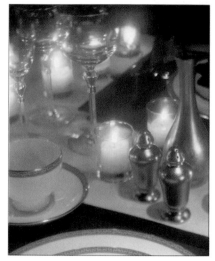

■ **Reward yourself** *once you have reached a milestone. Make it a special occasion. Set the table, add flowers and candles, and enjoy yourself.*

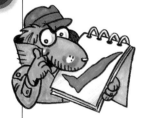

In France, where food is king but the natives are slim, ice cream is among the best in the world. But when you order a scoop, it's about the size of a golf ball, compared to the tennis ball giants in the United States. So if you want to enjoy la glace the French way, buy a melon baller and use it as a scoop.

At the supermarket

FOOD SHOPPING CAN *make or break your diet. If you do it the right way, it can be a major diet aid. Think of it this way: If you don't buy it, you can't eat it. Make a shopping list before every trip to the store and do not buy anything that's not on your list. Look back at the scavenger hunt you went on in Chapter 11. The lower-calorie foods you found can form the basis of your list. Your daily or weekly menus are the contents.*

Once you get to the market, be sure to read the label of everything you plan to buy. Look at per-serving calorie counts, fat and sugar content, and keep an eye out for hidden trans fats.

Spend time exploring the produce department. Fresh fruits and vegetables are your best friends. They are excellent sources of complex carbohydrates. They tend to be high-bulk, low calorie-density foods. They add color, variety, and interest to meals. They are refreshing. They provide a wide range of textures. They are excellent snack foods. Make a quick detour when you get to the candy, cookie, and baked goods aisle. There is nothing there that you need.

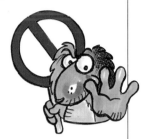

Whatever you do, never shop on an empty stomach. There's nothing like being hungry to tempt you into foolish purchases.

You and your refrigerator

FOR MOST PEOPLE, *the refrigerator is "ground zero" in the war against overweight. That's where the food is, making it the most dangerous spot in the house. Short of putting a lock on it and hiding the key, what can you do to make your refrigerator safer?*

Clean it out

On the eve of beginning your diet, take everything out of the refrigerator and freezer and get rid of anything you know will cause trouble. Double fudge pecan swirl ice cream? Toss it. Chocolate syrup? Give it to your neighbor. Whipping cream? Give it to the cat. Maraschino cherries? You won't be making ice cream sundaes so you don't need them. You get the idea. Every refrigerator has its own "regulars" that should be banished. Take a look at what's in yours and do some serious triage. Maybe it's leftover pizza or sour cream clam dip, maybe it's a lifetime supply of jams and jellies or cold meatloaf or a container of creamy cole slaw. Whatever it is, it's all got to go!

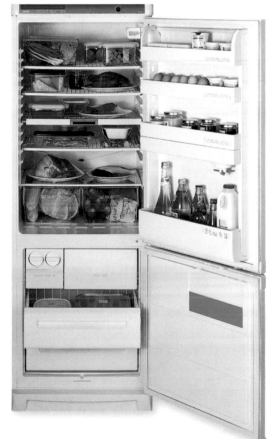

■ **Reorganize** *your refrigerator thoroughly. Sort through every compartment, removing anything that spells danger to your diet.*

Take inventory

Make a list of everything that survived the cut and tape it to the door. Every time you add something, write it on the list. And every time you make a withdrawal, note that on the list. Stopping to write things down is a good way to make you more mindful of what you do with what's in the fridge.

Rearrange the contents

Now it's time to put things back in the refrigerator, but arrange them strategically. If you're in the habit of opening the door and grabbing the first thing that catches your eye, make that thing something you can eat without doing too much damage. If you had to leave some high-calorie items (for the sake of others in your family or for other practical reasons), make them hard to reach. For example:

a) In the freezer, put the ice cream behind the ice cubes.

b) A pitcher of water should be front and center, and the bottle of fruit punch in the back.

c) Butter is better on a lower shelf. The same goes for cheese, cold cuts, and other fatty foods.

d) Leftovers, if you must have them, should be kept in tightly closed containers. (It's just too easy to reach for a morsel in an open dish or one that is lightly draped with clear plastic wrap.)

e) Pride of place should go to fruits and vegetables: If they're easy to get at, you'll reach for them first.

Never eat while standing in front of an open fridge. Not even just for a taste or to "check" if something is still fresh and edible.

If you plan to eat something, open the door, take out the food or ingredients, close the door, and set the food down on a table or counter. Prepare it, put it on a plate, bring the plate to another room, sit down, and then – and only then – dig in. If you cannot wait to go through these steps, that's a sure sign you have a problem.

Try to break the habit through mindfulness. If that does not work, talk with your doctor or other professional, join a support group, and focus on conquering your eating compulsion.

Decorate it

Get yourself some refrigerator magnets and turn the door into a weight-loss bulletin board. Post your inventory withdrawal and deposit list, and a revolving array of the goals and positive changes you put on index cards in Chapter 15. Add some photos you clipped from magazines of bodies you'd like to call your own. If you prefer, put up cartoons and anything else that will lighten your mood and keep you motivated.

Do it again

Especially if you live with other people, your refrigerator is an evolving creature. It's a good idea to repeat the pruning, inventory, and rearrangement on a regular basis. You may need to do it once a week or may be able to make it a monthly routine. Whenever it starts looking like a minefield again, get in there and defuse it.

A simple summary

✓ Keeping a food diary continues to be essential. It will keep you honest and focused.

✓ Mindfulness means being aware of when, what, and why you are eating. It is an important behavior-modification technique.

✓ Plan everything you eat and eat nothing you have not planned.

✓ Learn to recognize a serving on your plate and exercise portion control at every meal.

✓ Let true physiological hunger be your guide to when you start and when you stop eating.

✓ Cravings are the product of psychological rather than physiological hunger. Fight them with behavior modification, not with food.

✓ Learn to be a careful shopper. Keep the Trojan horse out of your shopping cart and it won't get into your kitchen.

✓ On the eve of the beginning of your diet, renovate and redecorate your refrigerator to keep it from being the most dangerous place in your house. Throw away anything you know is going to cause trouble

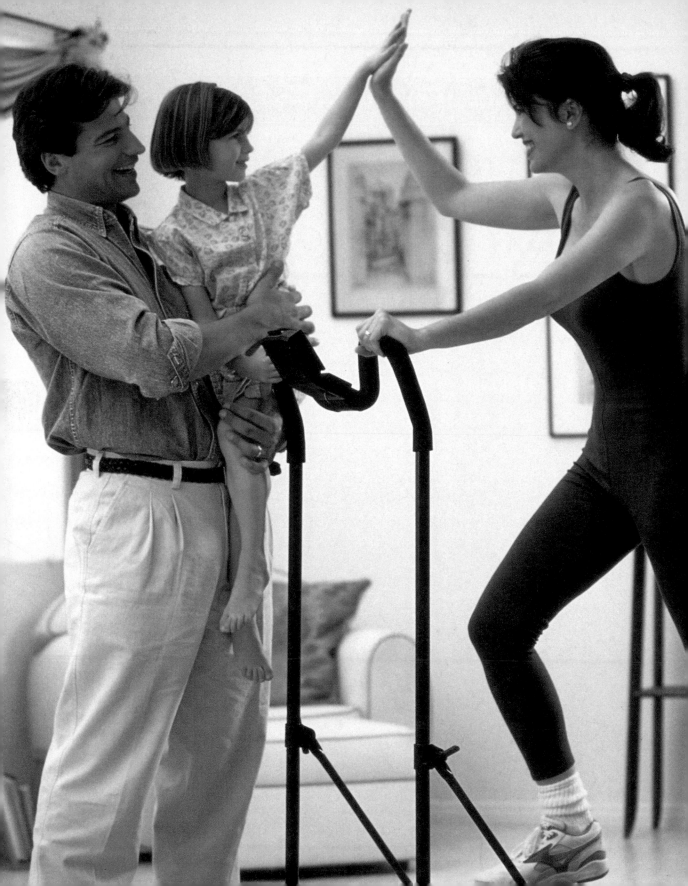

Chapter 17

Living With Your Exercise Routine

Your EXERCISE ROUTINE travels hand in hand with your weight-loss diet. That partnership is what will make the whole thing work. Unlike dieting, exercising for weight loss is something you do instead of not doing. It will keep your spirit buoyed at a time when you might otherwise feel deprived. Still, being more active involves making changes, and that takes time, persistence, and patience. This chapter will help you make those changes in a positive and fun-filled way.

In this chapter...

✓ Dedicate time to be active

✓ Simply keep it interesting

✓ Keep it safe

✓ Starting over

✓ Exercise extras

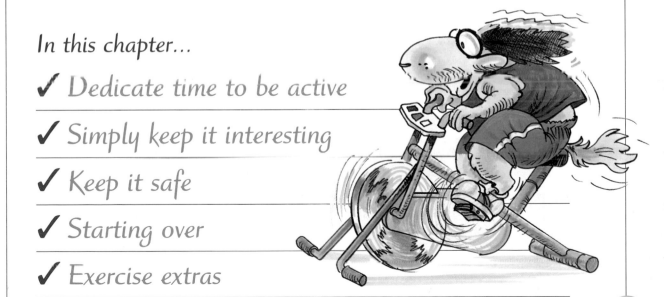

Dedicate time to be active

ACTIVITY SHOULD BE MORE *than an afterthought, something you do after you've done everything else. If you put it last on your list of to-dos or think of it as optional, chances are you'll never get to it. Instead, make activity an essential part of your day. Like eating, brushing your teeth, and other personal grooming activities, exercise is a must. Socializing, watching television, and shopping are the extras.*

Make sure you schedule a specific block of time for activity.

Decide in advance what you will do each day and set aside a time for it. Write it on your calendar or in your appointment book, and don't cancel out. When scheduling exercise, the obvious choice is some time that is "free." After school, after work, and on the weekends are popular choices.

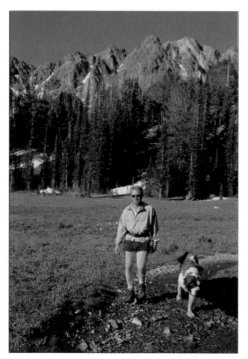

■ **If you like walking,** *schedule in a hike at a beauty spot over the weekend. Exercising in stunning scenery may help inspire you and spur you on in your fitness campaign.*

Turn dangerous times of day to your advantage by scheduling an exercise session for a time when you tend to act or eat irresponsibly.

For example, if the middle of the afternoon is a low-energy time for you and you usually spend it watching daytime television or zoning out at your desk, pick yourself up and take a walk or an aerobics class instead. If you fill your evenings by filling your stomach, get out of the house, away from the refrigerator, and go dancing. Not a morning person? Maybe a wake-up swim or stretching session will get you ready for the rest of the day.

Take a look at both your food and activity diaries and see if there are "dead spots" in your day. It may sound backward, but times when your energy is at its lowest are exactly the times when you should be doing something active. Energy feeds energy.

These periods of low energy indicate that your metabolism is slowing. Remember the best, safest, and most natural way to rev up your metabolism? That's right: by exercising.

Get specific

Take out your weight-loss notebook and start a new page titled "My Exercise Schedule" and date it. Leave space for revision, since you will want to review and make changes as time passes.

Divide the page lengthwise into three columns. Label one "Goals," the second "Means," and the third "Notes." Begin by filling in the goals; add a timetable for each one. The goal is a long-term one; the timetable will contain the steps you'll take to get there, which are short-term goals. You might want to highlight the long-term and short-term goals in different colors.

Next, fill in the means: specific exercises or activities you will do on a daily basis. You can plan it as a one- or two-week chunk. Finally, make notes about information, assistance, and equipment you'll need. Add anything else you want to keep in mind as you embark on this program.

Don't get hung up on the details. If you're not sure exactly what your goals should be, write down a general idea. If you're not sure what a reasonable time period is, make an estimate and give yourself permission to change the dates as you go along. The idea is to sketch out a plan, not to hand down a life sentence.

On the next page is a sample notebook page. Your goals and specific plans will probably be different and you may prefer to organize your page in another way. Do it however it makes sense to you.

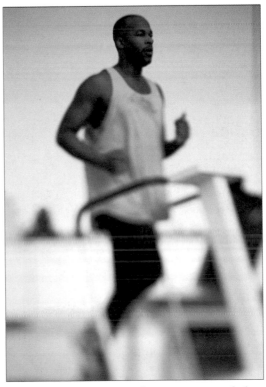

■ **When planning specific exercises,** *include more than one option for each day so weather and other obstacles won't give you the excuse to abandon a session.*

My exercise schedule

August 8

Goals	Means	Notes
Greater flexibility so I don't get leg cramps when I walk fast or run, and don't feel so stiff. Timetable: 3 months Increase arm and leg reach by 3 inches without pain.	15 minutes of stretches every morning before breakfast; stretches before every exercise session; get up from desk and stretch 5 minutes mid-morning, mid-afternoon.	Get info on stretches; get stretching video.
Stronger arms: be able to do three sets of 12 reps with 8-pound weights. Timetable: 6 months Start with one set @ 2 pounds; increase sets each week at each level, stabilize for 1 week, then increase weight by 1 pound.	Strength training 3x/week: Monday, Wednesday, Friday.	Get set of weights (2, 3, 5 lb) Check with trainer at gym, friends, magazines, for good lifting moves.
Better endurance: be able to run a mile without feeling like I'm dying: 7-minute mile? Timetable: 9 months Walk/run for 15 minutes 1x/week; add a minute each week for a month; then 2x/week for a month; then increase run, decrease walk until it's all run; then begin to measure distance and increase speed.	Walk/run Saturday morning; add Tuesday evening before dinner after first month. Stair climb when weather is bad.	Don't worry about speed or distance until I can comfortably run 30 minutes 2x/week; find indoor running track when weather is bad? Join a running club? Do it with a friend? Get good running shoes! Remember to stretch/warm up/cool down.

■ **This exercise** *plan sets out three long-term goals (in pink type) that the writer wants to achieve within a given timetable. The short-term goals (in red type), means, and notes are the routes to success.*

Keep your diary

Once you have this outline, make a weekly schedule using the activity diary blank at the back of this book or write it on your appointment calendar. Each time you keep your appointment, check it off. If you don't keep it, or if you do less (or more?), make a note of that, along with the reason for the change. Was it the weather? Give yourself more choices so heat, rain, snow, or other climate issues don't sideline you. Were you feeling unwell? Get back to your routine as quickly as you can. Is it taking too much time? Try to schedule shorter but more frequent sessions. If you have other explanations or excuses, check out Chapter 19 to learn how to troubleshoot your activity plan.

Finally, review your plan periodically. You may be doing better than you planned or you may be falling short. It may be necessary to reset your short term goals or change your means.

Simply keep it interesting

THERE ARE 7 DAYS IN EVERY WEEK, *and you should do something active on every one of them. That does not mean it should always be the same thing. In fact, it definitely should not. Even people who are training for a marathon don't make the same run every day.*

Vary your activities to stave off boredom. Go to the gym for strength training one day and play some sports the next. Have a bike ride or skate with friends or family the next day. The following day you might return to the gym, but take a class instead of working solo. Plan evening activities like bowling or dancing. Make weekends the time for physical fun.

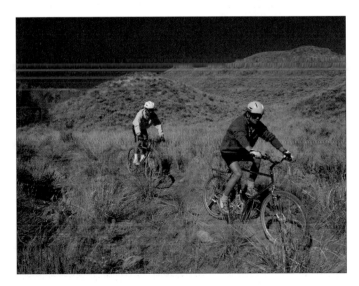

■ **Vary your route,** *try different activities, and make your exercise schedule enjoyable so that you stay on track.*

It is particularly important to vary the type of activity to avoid overdoing it.

Lifting weights day after day is a bad idea. Your muscles need time to recover, so it is recommended that you take at least one day off between strength-training sessions. Since strength training is an anaerobic activity, alternate with an aerobic one: A step or *low-impact aerobics* class is ideal.

Exercise with the seasons

Keep the weather in mind when you schedule your activities. Working out indoors is a good idea when it's very hot or very cold.

If you do exercise outdoors in extremely hot or cold weather, start at a low intensity and then gradually increase it. Warm-ups are especially important at temperature extremes. And when it is hot, be sure to drink lots of water and protect yourself from the sun.

Use seasonal change as an advantage. You can add interest to your walk, run, ride, or skate by doing it on a colorful fall day. Water sports and hot weather are a refreshing combination. And the rebirth of spring can inspire you to turn over a new leaf yourself.

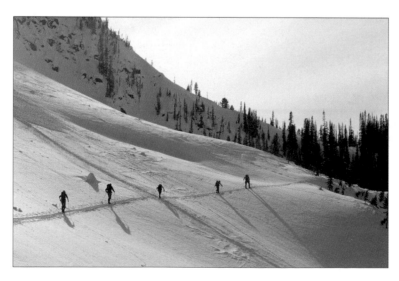

■ **Winter sports** *provide a perfect opportunity to be outdoors in beautiful surroundings when more sedentary types would find it too cold.*

Challenge yourself

One of the best ways to keep it interesting is to present yourself with new challenges. Make each activity session a contest. Can you do it a bit longer, farther, faster, higher?

Pushing yourself is a good way to measure how far you've progressed. Staying with the status quo is the quickest way to boredom.

Try to add on something periodically. You can do it each session, or once a week, or after a particular move, exercise, or effort has become easy. Keep track of any incremental improvements you make by writing them in your notebook.

After you've been exercising for a while, you may feel comfortable enough to join a team or other group. Competition with others is a way to challenge yourself, but it may not be for everybody. Give it a try, though. If you find it adds interest and motivation, keep it up. If not, return to solo or noncompetitive pursuits without being critical of yourself.

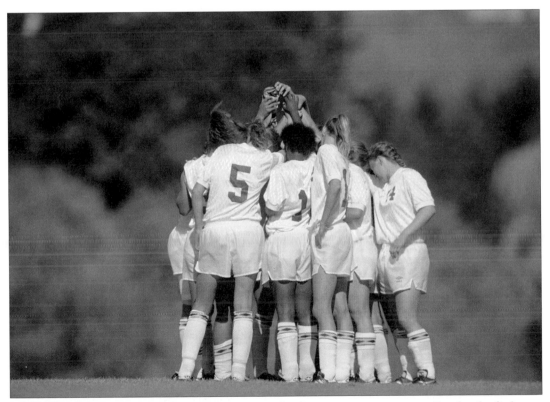

■ **Playing a team sport** *can be a great fun, especially if you're a competitive type. People who find running on a treadmill excruciatingly difficult will often race around a sports field without flagging as they get caught up in the excitement of the game.*

Keep it safe

IF YOU ARE VERY OVERWEIGHT *or have been inactive for a long time, beginning to be more active should be a gradual process. Don't start without talking to your doctor about your current state of health and fitness and your plans for improving both. Even if you are not seriously out of shape, taking it slowly is the safe way to go.*

Don't overdo it. I'm hoping all this talk about exercise will make you gung-ho, but I don't want you to give up in the early days because you are a mass of aches and pains.

The right equipment

Many of the activities you have to choose from require little or nothing in the way of special equipment. Still, there are some basics. You should have some workout and exercise clothes that keep you warm and dry in wet and cold weather, but are breathable so your sweat will "wick" away. A pair of well-fitting and supportive shoes is a must. They should have no-slip soles and should not be so worn out that they won't absorb shocks or will put you off balance. If you use other equipment – whether it's a stationary or moving bicycle, skates, weights, treadmills and stair climbers, racquets, bat, balls, whatever – they should be sturdy and in good repair. If you're just starting out and want to give an activity a try, borrow the equipment or use it in a public or commercial facility.

Warm up/cool down

The two most important parts of any exercise come at the beginning and the end. I'm sorry to say that they are also two things most often omitted. Warming up and cooling down help your body adjust to the change of pace that activity entails. Your muscles and your heart and lungs have to gradually get up to speed. And when they are speeding, they shouldn't stop cold. Immediate pain and morning-after soreness will result if you don't take the time to warm up and cool down.

Warming up literally increases the temperature of your muscles by directing more blood to them. "Warm muscles" extend and contract more quickly than muscles that are cold, preventing strain and cramping. Warming up also increases the flow of blood to your coronary arteries and lungs, which will be working hard during your exercise. The cool-down allows your breathing to return to normal and your heart rate to come down gradually from at or near your THR to close to your RHR. It also gently redirects blood from your muscles to a more even distribution around your body.

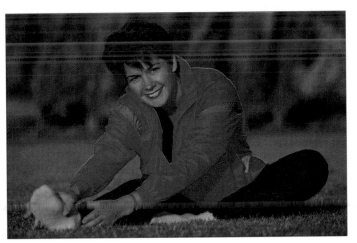

■ **When working out** *on your own, allow a minimum of 10 minutes to warm up before exercising, and at least 5 minutes to cool down.*

Any decent exercise class will include warming up and cooling down. If you find yourself in one that does not, talk to the instructor and if there is no improvement, change classes. As an alternative, start early and do your own warm-up and stay on to cool down.

When you are working out on your own, it's up to you. Warm up for at least 10 minutes, keeping it at low to moderate intensity. The best warm-up uses the same muscles your activity will. So if you will be running, start by running lightly in place, or walking and gradually increasing your pace before you break into a run. Swing your arms, flex your feet and knees.

Don't forget to breathe when warming up and cooling down. Your body needs extra oxygen, and it needs to rid itself of carbon dioxide and other toxins. So keep the air going in and out. Your cool-down can be shorter than your warm up, but it should be no less than 5 minutes. Gradually decrease the intensity of whatever you are doing. Let your breathing and heart beat return to normal.

Stretching

Stretching can be part of warming up and cooling down or an exercise activity in itself. It is an excellent choice for people who are very overweight, who have been inactive, who are elderly, pregnant, or for other reasons need to exercise gently. Many gyms and health clubs have stretching classes, and there are stretching videos galore. Some exercise techniques emphasize stretching. For example, most yoga postures involve gently stretching specific parts of the body and holding the stretch while breathing.

INTERNET

www.learn2.com/05/ 0503/0503.asp

At this web page, you'll find an animated series of stretches that shows you exactly how to do it.

Even if stretching is not the focus of your activity or routine, it should be a part of it.

Starting over

YOU'VE MISSED SOME OF YOUR EXERCISE *appointments. What do you do? If it's been a day or two, just jump back in. If it's been a week or more, you'll have to go back a few steps and get back in shape. This may mean resetting some short-term goals. It should also mean looking at the reasons for the lapse.*

Were you too busy? Were you really, or did you give priority to something else? Remember how important activity is to your plan and to your present and future health. Was it the weather? Check your list of options.

Whatever the reason for allowing your exercising to lapse, the most important thing is to get back into action as soon as you can.

Don't let a lapse of a day or so turn into a return to the land of the couch potato. You've worked too hard to let it slide. Being active gives you an emotional boost. That means that dropping activity has probably left you feeling low, maybe depressed. That can be the beginning of a vicious cycle: Depression feeds low self-esteem and a general feeling of defeat. The best thing you can do to fight this web of negativism is to get moving.

When you're forced to stop

Sometimes you simply have to take a break from your exercise routine. If you feel sick or have been injured, keeping up with daily exercise may not be possible. If the break was just for a few days or a week at most, you can get back into action without any special precautions. The important thing is to do it, and as soon as possible.

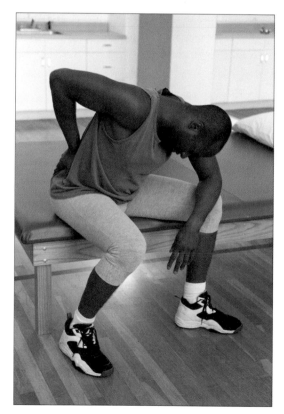

■ **An injury** *may mean that you have to adjust the type and intensity of your exercise. Always seek your doctor's advice.*

292

After an injury

If you hurt yourself, either during exercise or in some other way, how much you can exercise and how soon are matters to discuss with a doctor. If your injury is not serious enough to require medical attention, it's probably not serious enough to cause a break in your routine. If it's a matter of muscle soreness from a workout that was too vigorous or that did not begin and end with stretching, do something different the next day or two and return to the offending activity with new resolve. Instead of strength training, take a walk or bike ride, or try yoga. When you go back to the weights, be sure to stretch. Start with lighter weights and fewer sets and then gradually work your way back up to where you were.

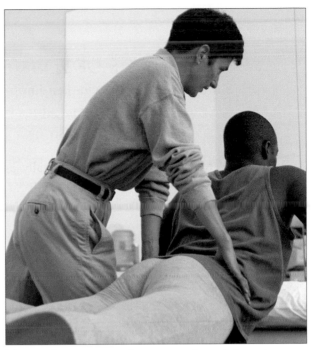

■ **Your doctor may** *refer you to a physical therapist or other professional to help you get back in shape and avoid a similar injury in future.*

Exercise and back pain

Back pain need not be a reason to stop or never even begin to exercise. The most common type of back pain is in the lower back. It is often caused or worsened by weak abdominal muscles, which shift the burden of carrying the weight to the back. Exercise that strengthens the abdominals will also relieve this kind of back pain.

A study of people with low back pain found that those who took exercise classes that included strengthening exercises for all main muscle groups, stretching exercises, a relaxation session, and brief education on back care experienced significantly less pain over the long term and missed fewer days of work than those who did not exercise.

The study stressed that people with low back pain should return to normal activity as soon as possible, but that exercise should be done under the direction of someone trained in exercise physiology.

Exercise extras

UNLESS YOU ARE BEDRIDDEN, *you are more or less active all day long. There are a lot of exercise extras built into your day, and you can add more with a little thought and not much more effort. Think of these as "snacks in reverse." When you take a nibble of something extra, you are adding calories. When you do something in the course of your normal day, you are subtracting them.*

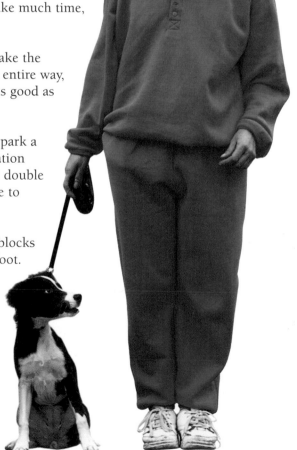

Here are some exercise extras that won't take much time, but will burn calories:

a Instead of the elevator or escalator, take the stairs. You don't have to walk up the entire way, but walking up one flight or two is as good as a few minutes on a Stairmaster.

b Park and walk. If you're in your car, park a block or two away from your destination and walk the rest of the way. You get double for your money since you'll also have to walk back.

c Get off the bus too soon. Add a few blocks to your journey home, but do it on foot.

d Walk while you talk. Whenever you're on the phone, walk around the room instead of sitting down. With a long cord or a cordless phone, there's no reason to be desk-bound.

■ **If you have a dog,** *make it your job to exercise him or her, or tag along.*

(e) Walk your children to or from school, or do it on bikes or skates.

(f) Volunteer for active chores. Anything that requires reaching, lifting, pushing, pulling, or running up and down the stairs is an exercise extra. If mowing the lawn, vacuuming, mopping the floor, dusting high shelves, and cleaning the garage or attic are up for grabs in your household, be the one who signs up for these tasks and leave washing dishes, ironing, and folding laundry for someone else.

A simple summary

✔ Set aside a specific time of day, every day, for some kind of activity.

✔ Keep track of your fitness goals and the means by which you want to achieve them.

✔ Variety is the spice of an active life. Keep your interest high by varying the time, place, and type of exercise you choose.

✔ Safety first: Make sure you have the right clothes and equipment for anything you choose to do.

✔ Check with a doctor if you haven't exercised in a long time or if your health might limit what and how much you do.

✔ Don't forget to add a warm-up, cool-down, and stretch to everything you do.

✔ If you're starting over after a break in your routine, gradually work your way up to where you were when you stopped.

✔ Engage in "snacking in reverse" by cramming as many exercise extras as possible into your day.

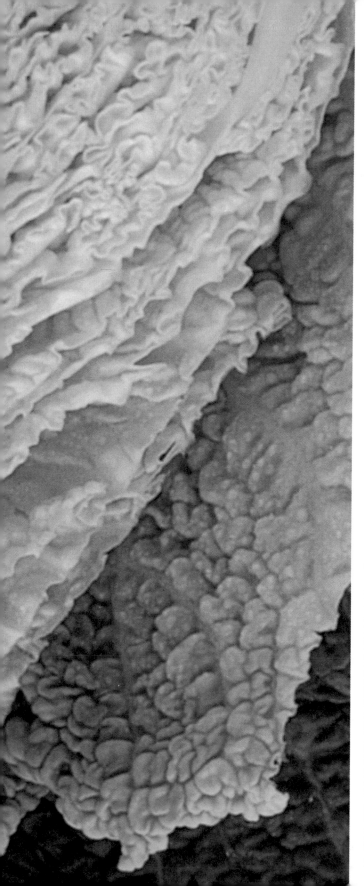

PART SIX

LEAFY GREEN VEGETABLES ARE FULL OF NUTRIENTS

Keeping It Up

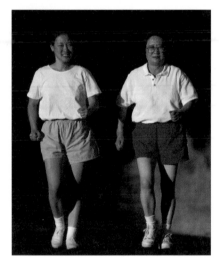

THE MOST EFFECTIVE weight-loss *plan* relies on modifying behavior: replacing the habits that made you overweight with habits that will keep you fit and trim. But old habits die hard and it takes time to make new ones. This is a transition period, a time when you are subject to many *challenges*.

In this part of the book, you'll find helpful strategies to tackle these challenges head-on, from dealing with the weight-loss plateau through *surviving* the holidays without abandoning your diet and troubleshooting your exercise routine. Finally, you'll learn how to make the transition from weight loss to weight *maintenance* and adjust to changes as you grow older. Above all, the emphasis is on staying active as the best weight-loss plan of all.

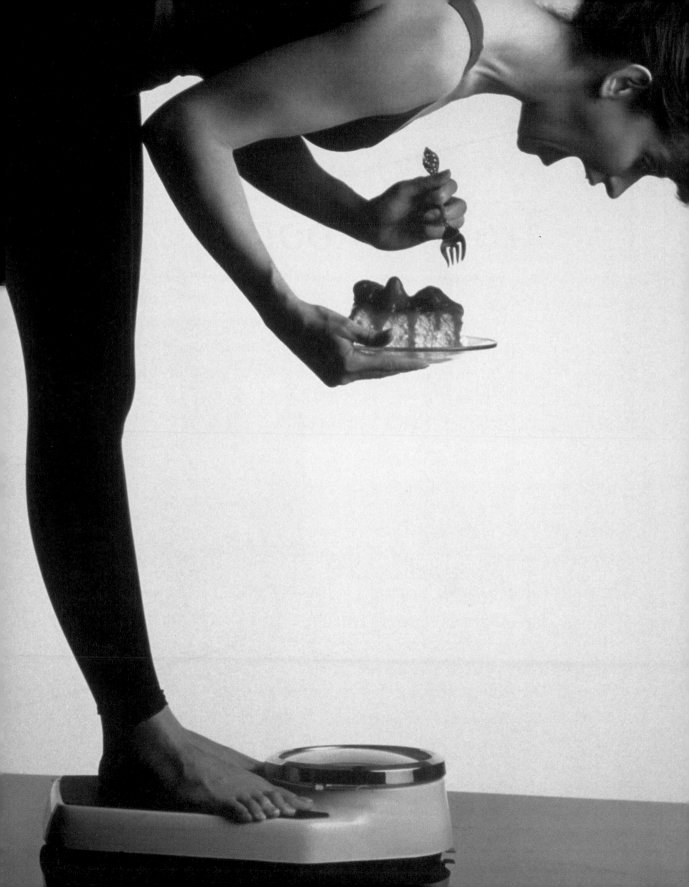

Chapter 18

Diet Troubleshooting

IF DIETING WERE EASY, none of us would be overweight. Hunger, cravings, and the magnet of old habits make day-to-day living with a diet a lot like walking across a minefield. Can you make it to the end of the day without a misstep? You can if you adopt the helpful strategies for tackling these challenges in the pages that follow.

In this chapter...

✓ I'm stuck on a plateau

✓ I'm having a snack attack!

✓ I've got a sweet tooth ache

✓ I get the midnight munchies

✓ I'm dreading eating out

✓ It's party time

✓ I've lapsed

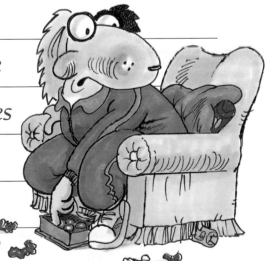

I'm stuck on a plateau

YOUR WEIGHT-LOSS DIET STARTED OUT JUST FINE. You lost a few pounds in the first month, then the loss slowed down. It's been 4 months now and things have ground to a halt. You are frustrated and wonder what's going on. In all likelihood you've hit the fabled weight-loss plateau. But before you settle on that explanation, let's look a little deeper.

Revising your goal

How close are you to your normal weight? Take a look at the height-weight table in Chapter 1. Are you near or even at what is considered normal for you? Recalculate your BMI. Are you in the range of healthy weight – 24.9 or below? Maybe you've lost enough. You may want to lose 10 or more pounds to get to your goal, but now's the time to ask if that goal is realistic. You've done a great job. Perhaps you should shift into maintenance mode and concentrate on not gaining, rather than on losing more weight.

Are you cheating?

You may claim – and even truly believe – that you are not exceeding your planned daily calorie intake, but you may be fooling yourself. Take a look at your daily food diary. Have you been keeping it faithfully? Have you written down everything you've eaten? Or are you beginning to slip by forgetting the handful of M&Ms, the sip of your friend's beer, the sample of sauce while you're cooking, the forkful of pie from your spouse's slice?

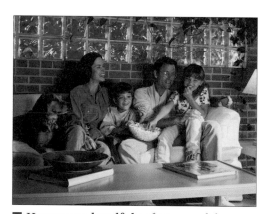

■ **How many handfuls** *of popcorn did you really eat while watching a movie with your family? Keeping up your food diary will help you avoid careless eating.*

Small sips and bitty bites can add up to a lot of calories. If you have kitchen duties, you are at higher risk for careless and unconscious eating.

As the cook, you probably do a fair amount of tasting during preparation. If you clean up, you may eat the last morsel before scraping the plate, or finish off leftovers too small to be worth keeping. Avoid these tidbits if you can, and if you can't, write them down in your food diary.

Before you make any changes, spend a week keeping your diary scrupulously. Add up your total intake every day. See what the numbers say.

Simply reset your set point

If your numbers check out and you still want to lose, you have three choices: You can eat less, exercise more, or try a combination of the two.

The most effective, and probably most pleasurable way to reset your set point is to increase your level of activity.

INTERNET

www.thriveonline.com/
weight/habits/week2.
html

A new food diary might rekindle your interest in keeping track. (Kind of like a new outfit or a new pair of shoes.) You'll find a printable one at this web site.

Resetting your set point to increase activity will not only burn calories; it will also increase your metabolic rate and thereby maximize the "burn." This is the most efficient way to reset your set point, that place where intake and output seem to be in balance so you neither gain nor lose weight.

To add time, frequency, or intensity to your daily activity, try the following:

1. Do one more set or increase the weight you lift by a pound.

2. Walk 10 minutes longer or run just a bit faster.

3. Add 15 minutes to your workout or a few laps to your swim.

4. Move up to a more advanced class.

5. Replace a low-intensity activity with one that is more challenging.

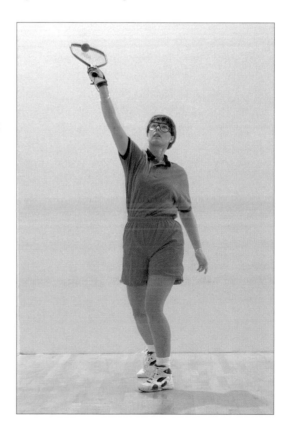

■ **The best way to move** *off that weight-loss plateau is to rev up your metabolic rate by raising your level of exercise. Move up a gear by putting in a little extra time or increasing the intensity of your program.*

I'm having a snack attack!

IT HAPPENS TO THE BEST OF US. *Real hunger, boredom, temptation, circumstances conspire to bring us up close and personal with a bag of potato chips or a bowl of jelly beans. We're between meals and we know we shouldn't, but . . .*

Safe snacking

Snacking need not be dangerous. If you do it furtively, desperately, in a state of denial, you may find yourself with cake crumbs on your chin before you know what hit you. If you plan for snacks, you can have a supply of healthful choices from which to choose.

SOME SAFE SNACKING IDEAS

When you've just got to have something, try the following healthful ideas:

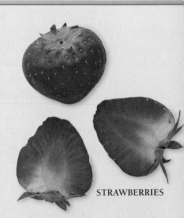
STRAWBERRIES

1. Fresh fruit: Apple, pear, banana, orange, tangerine, pineapple, peach, melon, grapes, berries.

2. Slide chunks of fruit on a wooden skewer and sprinkle with sesame seeds.

3. Spread slices of fruit with a thin layer of peanut butter.

4. Want an icy refreshing treat? Try frozen grapes, or puree fruit in a blender and pour into ice-cube trays; insert a toothpick in each one.

5. Raw vegetables: Carrots, celery, cucumber, cherry tomatoes, sweet peppers, radishes, broccoli and cauliflower florets, and more. Sliced or cubed and chilled, these are refreshing on their own. Or, dip them into salsa or yogurt spiced with chili or curry powder or a bit of barbecue sauce. You can also chop them fine and add some tomato juice and a dash of hot sauce for a cup of instant gazpacho.

CHERRY TOMATOES

Any food can be a snack if you eat it in snack-sized portions; too much of any "snack food" can turn into a meal.

It all comes down to calories. One cookie is a snack; six is a mistake. The same goes for an ounce of cheese on three or four crackers versus a half-pound chunk and a boxful.

Don't get blindsided by the yen to snack. Have a supply of safe snacks on hand. These should be low-calorie, high-bulk items that are quick and easy to prepare, if they need any preparation at all. They should have interesting textures too.

INTERNET

www.phys.com/
b_nutrition/02solutions/
04snacko/snacko_
detect.htm

Got a yen for something spicy? Here you'll find a list of snack ideas. Choose one and get a rating from good through so-so to bad and find out the calorie and fat content.

6 Dried fruit: Apricots, raisins, dates, figs, prunes, cherries, and more. These are sweet and full of fiber, but also higher in calories than fresh fruit. A little goes a long way in staving off hunger.

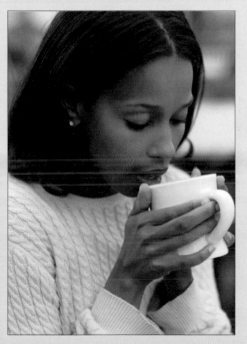

7 Pickles, olives, and other preserved vegetables add zip to any snack.

8 Rice cakes, air-popped corn, pretzels, breadsticks: They pack the crunch of chips without any of the fat.

9 Bouillon or consommé: A cup or bowl of something warm and flavorful, without the calories of full-blown soup. Or stir in some gelatin and chill for an elegant gelée.

10 Diet soft drinks, including flavored seltzers.

Surely you can think of others. Make a list and keep them on hand when you simply can't wait for the next meal.

■ **Coffee and tea,** *hot or iced, are good safe "snack" ideas.*

Plan for that snack

When you plan your daily menus, assume that you will want some snacks and build them into the plan. Find out the per-serving calorie count of various snacks and add them to your expected daily total. But remember: You can always eat less than a serving. If you don't end up having that snack, all the better, but if you do, those calories will be in your budget.

Practice mindful snacking. Stop what you are doing and concentrate on your snack. Measure or weigh out a serving and put it on a plate or in a bowl.

Put the package or container away. Give yourself a set period of time for the snack. This is a 10-minute break, for example. You will do nothing during that time except for having the snack, and when the 10 minutes are over, so is the eating.

I've got a sweet tooth ache

THERE'S SOMETHING ABOUT SWEETS *few people can resist. If that's what you crave, nothing else will satisfy. You can pack in a lot of calories eating around a desire for sweets, so it's better to just go for it.*

Don't hold off until you're dying for a sweet.

If you keep fighting the desire for a sweet, you end up throwing caution to the winds and regretting it as soon as you've downed the last bon-bon. Instead, make a list of safe sweets and keep some on hand.

a Sugar substitutes, used in moderation, will satisfy most urges. Diet sodas and candies, sugar-free puddings and cookies are all possibilities. Be sure to check the calorie content before you go wild. Sugar-free does not automatically equal low-calorie.

■ **If you can't overcome** *a sweet craving, it's better to have a candy than to keep denying yourself. Take one and then put away the jar!*

b Fresh fruits are naturally sweet foods and most are low-calorie choices. They're a good source of vitamins and fiber, and they offer a lot of variety in texture. Smooth bananas, crunchy apples, refreshing melons, tangy grapefruits are all good ways to sweeten your day.

c Try some fruit gelatin or applesauce. These low-calorie sweets can be dessert or an energy pick-me-up. You can even find sugar-free versions of both.

d If nothing but the "real thing" will satisfy you, have your sweet, but have just a little. A mini-scoop of ice cream can feel like a treat. Pick a flavor you dream about, serve it with a melon baller, put it in an elegant wineglass, and eat it with a demitasse spoon. And before you sit down to this indulgence, put the carton back in the freezer.

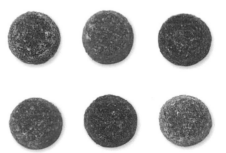

e Add it up and write it down. If you have a slice of cake, it will cost you, but you may decide it's worth the price. As long as your calorie intake does not exceed your daily goal, you're doing all right. Be sure to write down the mood, trigger, and circumstance that led you to that cake. It may help you fight the urge another day.

■ **A ripe, creamy-fleshed banana** *contains plenty of sugar to satisfy that sweet craving, but is still low in calories. Bananas are also a good source of potassium.*

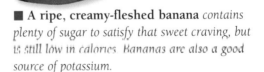

■ **No matter how little** *or how much you eat, make sure you include every sweet food in your daily total.*

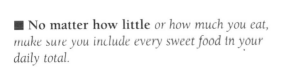

I get the midnight munchies

MIDNIGHT SNACKING *is rarely part of anyone's eating plan. It comes at a time when your metabolism is at its lowest ebb. You're tired and the cares of the day may be weighing on you heavily. If you've eaten dinner, you're probably not physiologically hungry. Indeed, the midnight munchies are a prime symptom of emotional hunger, and should be treated as such.*

The best thing to do when the munchies strike is to brush your teeth and go to sleep.

Fatigue will do the job if you don't have the energy to fight the attack. If you're not ready for bed but you've made a rule that the kitchen closes at 9 p.m., resist the urge to break it.

- Distract yourself with a book or television show
- Call up a friend and talk
- Put on some music and dance around the living room
- Do some stretches
- Practice some yoga postures to relax you and empty your mind

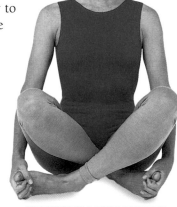

PRACTICING A YOGA POSTURE

In the belly of the beast

If you can't stay out of the kitchen, pour yourself a glass of water, pop a can of diet soda, or make a cup of caffeine-free tea to fill your stomach. If all else fails, have something to eat, but add the calories to your daily food diary and be sure to note the time, mood, and level of your hunger. If you have gone over your daily limit, try to make up for it the next day by eating less or exercising more.

If nighttime hunger is more than a sometime thing, incorporate it into your daily eating plan. Save some calories for bedtime and plan what you will eat. That way, the munchies won't get out of hand.

If you wake from sleep with a need to eat in the middle of the night, or if you consume most of your calories in the hours from midnight to dawn, consider the possibility that you suffer from night-eating syndrome (NES). Talk to your doctor about the problem.

I'm dreading eating out

WHEN YOU PLAN AND PREPARE your own meals, you can exercise control over your intake. It is considerably more challenging when you eat out, but it can be done. The most effective restaurant survival strategies begin before you open a menu.

1. Make it a special occasion. Try to limit your restaurant meals and enjoy the ones you have.

2. Plan ahead for eating out. Stay on the low-calorie side for the other meals that day so you have some extras to spend at the restaurant. Avoid impromptu restaurant meals, including last-minute decisions to grab a bite at the neighborhood eatery.

3. Choose restaurants that have low-calorie options. Seafood restaurants are a good choice, as are those specializing in cuisines that emphasize vegetables and grains, such as Chinese and other Asian, vegetarian, and natural foods.

4. Avoid fast-food emporiums and other restaurants that feature all-you-can-eat menus, buffets, and oversized meals.

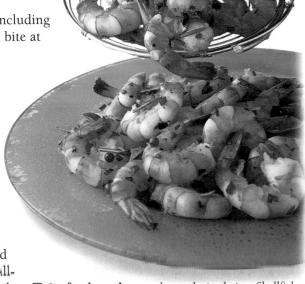

■ **Seafood meals** *are a low-calorie choice. Shellfish in particular are rich in iodine and zinc.*

5. Go with companions who support your diet; avoid anyone who is likely to tempt you with forbidden foods or urge you to "live it up, just this once."

Order wisely

Most restaurants these days cater to health-conscious diners. Many have low-fat selections, either as part of their regular offerings or as a separate dieter's menu. Many kitchens are willing to alter cooking and serving methods to suit special needs.

When ordering, start with a salad, soup, or fresh-fruit first course. This will take the edge off your hunger so you can eat what comes next slowly and in moderation. Don't be afraid to request:

a Fat-free or low-fat milk rather than whole milk or cream

b Gravy, sauce, and salad dressing on the side

c Butter-free vegetables

d Baked or boiled potatoes instead of french fries or mashed

e An extra vegetable

f Foods that are steamed, broiled, or poached rather than fried, sautéed, stewed, or braised

g An appetizer and soup or a salad rather than a main dish

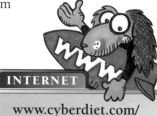

INTERNET

www.cyberdiet.com/
dining_out/restaurant
_choices.html

Here you'll find a list of cuisines and types of food as well as tips for finding "lite" dining choices on the menu of each.

Table manners

Once you've ordered the meal, drink a glass of water and talk with your companions. Enjoy the social aspects of the occasion. When the food arrives, eat it slowly. Savor every bite, but remember: You don't have to eat the whole thing. You can share with your dining companions or ask for a doggie bag. Don't treat the doggie bag as a midnight snack. Chances are it would make an excellent second dinner for you or another person the following day.

Don't even think about dessert until you've finished the main meal.

You may just want to skip dessert and have a cup of coffee while you wait for the check. Or order fresh fruit. At the most extreme, you can share a dessert with others at the table. A forkful of white chocolate souffle or tiramisu tastes just the same as a plateful. Trust me.

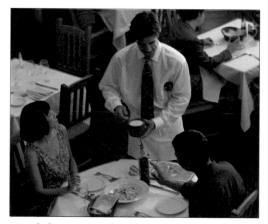

■ **While waiting** *for the food to come, push the breadbasket to far side of the table and ask the waiter to take the butter dish away.*

It's party time

WHETHER IT'S A SATURDAY NIGHT SOCIAL *or a weeklong string of holidays, gatherings that involve food are a dieter's nightmare. You don't want to miss out on the fun, but you also don't want to undo what you've accomplished.*

With a little planning, it is possible to make it through a dinner or cocktail party without torpedoing your weight-loss plan. You may even be able to survive the tricky territory that lies between Thanksgiving and New Year's.

Keep in mind that the best parties are about people, not about food.

Some strategies to help you out

Here are some ideas that will help you make it through any social occasion without wrecking your weight-loss program:

a Balance party meals with super low-calorie eating at home. If you know you'll be eating out later that day or even later that week, reduce the calories in every meal you can. Keep an eye on your weekly calorie intake.

b Be realistic. One meal won't make or break your diet, especially if you plan ahead. If you let your weight-loss plan ruin your fun, you may use this as an excuse to drop out. During the holidays, it may be more realistic to set a goal of not *gaining* weight than to expect to continue your loss.

c As soon as your coat's off, grab a low-cal beverage. If you really want alcohol, choose a wine spritzer and nurse it. A heavier drink will add calories (7 per gram, which can add up to 100 calories or more, depending on the size of the drink), and will loosen your inhibitions, including your resolve to eat wisely.

d Pass up the hors d'oeuvres. These tempting tidbits can add up to a full meal if you're not careful. Zero in on raw vegetables, but skip the dip.

e If it's a buffet, get at the end of the line so you're one of the last to sit down. Take a small plate, if possible, and go heavy on salads and complex carbohydrates. Do not, under any circumstances, go back for seconds.

f If it's a sit-down dinner, say no thank you to sauces, gravies, and anything else you know you should not eat. Ask for modest portions and don't be shy about leaving food on your plate. Second helpings are out.

(g) Talk to your companions. Enjoy the occasion. Focus on everything but the food. If the party includes dancing, games, or other activities, be sure to join in.

(h) After the meal, help with the clean up or go for a walk. Whatever you do, don't sit down. One of my favorite post-Thanksgiving dinner treats is a long walk I take with my cousins. We see each other rarely and it's a great opportunity to catch up on family news while digesting our turkey. And it sure beats dozing in front of the TV while pretending to watch the football games.

I've lapsed

OKAY, YOU HAD A MAJOR PIG-OUT, *you polished off the rest of the pizza, you ate all of the Valentine's chocolates in one sitting. You somehow managed to cram two days' worth of eating into a single 12-hour period. And you feel like a slob, a slug, a failure.*

Whatever you do, don't give up. Get back on the wagon and try again tomorrow. Don't let a lapse turn into an excuse to abandon your diet. Instead, turn it into a lesson.

What went wrong?

Ask yourself what caused the lapse. If you can identify the reasons for overindulging, it will help you avoid a next time.

(a) Was it a particular food? Add it to your black list and ban it from the house entirely. Throw out any that remains, never buy it again, and tell the friends of your diet to respect the ban.

(b) Did you have a hard day and need some comfort? Write about it in your journal. The next time you feel this way, try some stress-relieving exercise. Or make a list of non-food things that give you comfort: friends, a movie, music, a warm bath, flowers, whatever makes you feel special.

(c) Was it a particular person? Can you enlist this person as a friend of your diet or avoid him or her at times when you're vulnerable?

INTERNET

www.phys.com/general/index/weightloss.html

Look for "The Snack Bandit" under "Games." To use this fun, one-armed bandit, select a food, the number of helpings, and an activity, then pull the handle. Out will come how much of that activity is needed to burn off the calories. Did you know that you can eat a helping of Buffalo wings and pay for it with 49.93 minutes of aerobics?

Take the time to analyze the lapse. Try to trace the steps that led up to it. And then redouble your efforts to ensure you do not go down that road again.

Damage control

Happily, the calorie accountant takes a long view. Every day is a new day. If you ate too much today, you can make up for it tomorrow. If it was really bad, you might need two days or even a week. Figure out the calorie burden of your lapse. Divide by 300, for starters. Can you reduce your intake by 300 calories for as many days as it takes to pay off your debt? If that doesn't seem reasonable or likely, add some activity. Fifteen extra minutes will burn some calories and put you in a more positive frame of mind.

Above all, forgive yourself. You are only human and you are trying to do something very difficult: break old habits and establish healthier ones. This is not the work of a week or two; it's a lifelong pursuit.

A simple summary

✔ If your weight loss has come to a halt, it's time to reevaluate your goals, reexamine your compliance, and rev up your metabolism with more activity.

✔ The safest way to snack is to plan for it. Stay out of trouble by choosing low-calorie, satisfying snacks.

✔ Fight cravings for sweets with fruit or sugar free options.

✔ When the urge to eat comes at bedtime, go to sleep or find a way to distract yourself.

✔ When eating in restaurants, choose your venue carefully, order from the menu wisely, and carry home a doggie bag.

✔ Focus on the social aspects of a party and let food play second fiddle. Watch your alcohol intake so you don't end up ruining your resolve.

✔ A lapse is not a failure, so whatever you do, don't use it as an excuse to give up. Every day is a new day. Forgive the slip and rededicate yourself to your plan.

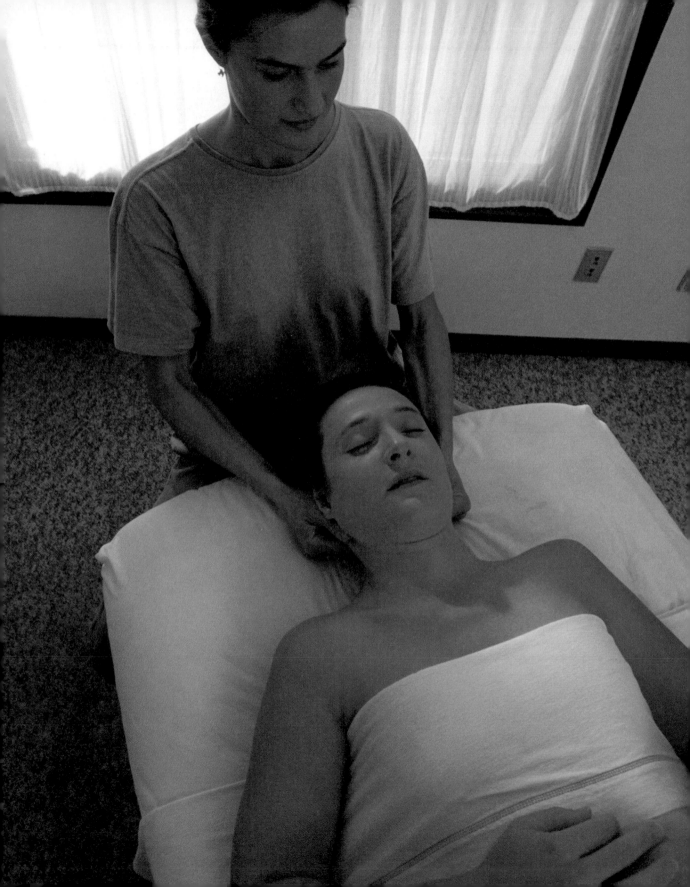

Chapter 19

Exercise Troubleshooting

I F YOU HAVE SPENT your adult life as a couch potato, becoming more active will take at least 6 months. You've set goals and made resolutions, but you will surely encounter roadblocks on your path to fitness. Here are some tips and strategies for overcoming common exercise problems.

In this chapter...

✓ It's boring

✓ It's too hard

✓ It takes too much time

✓ It hurts

✓ I've been sick

✓ It's simply too expensive

✓ I'll be away from home

✓ It doesn't seem to be working

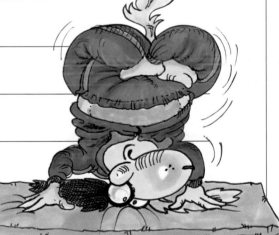

A PAMPERING TREATMENT AFTER AN EXERCISE SESSION CAN GIVE YOU A REAL BOOST

It's boring

IF YOU FIND EXERCISE BORING, *you've chosen the wrong kind. Activity is recreation, time off from the cares of the day. It should not be just another one of the things you have to do before you can enjoy yourself. It should be enjoyable in and of itself.*

If it has started to feel like the "same old same old," it's time for a change. If you've done your homework, your weight-loss notebook should have a list of the things you like to do. Retire some of your choices and make some new ones.

If there's nothing tempting on your list, take another look at the exercise options in Chapter 12. Check one of the many online sources that list activities and their calorie burns. Dial up the websites of particular sports and activities – from archery to yoga. Look into classes at your local Y or community center. Choose activities that will get you moving in a way that's fun.

a Enlist a friend to do it with you. That way you can combine socializing with exercising. Good conversation while you walk, run, skate, or bike will distract you from what feels like work. Making an unbreakable date will ensure that you really do it.

b Join a team. It's a great way to meet new people or spend time with folks you already know. A parent-child team adds quality time as well as providing an active role model for the next generation.

c If you are exercising alone, do it with music. A portable radio or tape/CD player is a lightweight exercise companion. If you choose upbeat music, it will help you maintain a lively tempo.

d Do it in an interesting place. From mall walking to mountain climbing, there's an environment that will strike your fancy. Try to combine your activity with something that interests you or engages a part of your mind other than the one that's counting reps.

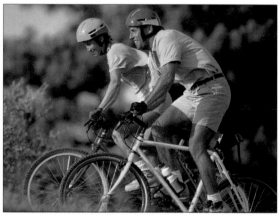

■ **If you find cycling** *on your own boring, go with a friend and choose an interesting route. An uphill climb will feel less like hard work if there's a stunning view.*

Add variety to whatever exercise you do.

Day after day of leg lifts will certainly be boring. Try to do something different every day and add something new at least once a month. This will keep you challenged in both body and mind.

Check your attitude

If you have kids or were one yourself, you know that the complaint, "It's boring" usually translates into "I don't wanna do it!" Is that what's going on with you?

If so, you may need to revisit or revise what's motivating you. Take out your weight-loss notebook and look at your motivators. Reminding yourself why you are doing this may be all it takes. Maybe you need to add some new motivators. If you want to get scared into action, go back and read Chapter 3 to find out what a life on the couch holds in store for you.

Call on the friends of your diet and tell them you're feeling stale. Ask them to give you a pep talk or make some suggestions. Ask them what they're doing this weekend, and if it's something active, invite yourself to go along.

It's too hard

IF EXERCISING MORE IS MAKING YOU TIRED *or sore, you may be overdoing it. That's not a reason to quit. Instead, take a step backward.*

1. Do fewer reps or fewer sets of whatever it is you are doing. If you are using weights, drop down by a pound or two. Then gradually work your way up. Add sets until it feels easy, and only then begin adding pounds.

2. If your activity involves speed, do it more slowly. Stay at that speed for at least a week, or longer if you still feel challenged.

3. If you're in a class that's more advanced than you are, look for one on more of a beginner's level. Or skip some moves. March or run in place while the rest of the class is doing triple-time reverse arabesques. (Don't worry, they're too busy to notice what you're doing.) Whatever you do, don't stop cold.

4. Take time off between exercise sessions. Do something else that uses different muscle groups or different parts of your body. Give yourself time to recover.

5 Check your equipment. Do your shoes absorb shocks and give you enough support? Are weight machines well lubricated and in good repair? Is your stationary bike, treadmill, stairclimber adjusted properly? You may be working harder than you should if you're fighting your equipment.

6 Are you getting enough rest? Are you drinking enough water? Are you exercising on an empty stomach? If an exercise session leaves you drained instead of energized, the "equipment" that needs adjustment may be you.

Finding an exercise that suits you

Give yourself the option to try something different. I am in awe of people who can live through a step class, but I know I am not one of them. My feet get tangled and I go left when everyone else goes right. I trip over the steps and find myself exhausted and confused. I have tried it for a while, but I know that, for me, it's just too hard. Fortunately, my gym offers a variety of classes throughout the day. I've found enough that are fun and at my level to keep me going there 3 days a week. Someday I may give stepping another try. Probably after I've mastered ocean kayaking and Himalayan trekking.

INTERNET

prevention.com/weight/ buzz/980722.buzz.html

Find out "How to make exercise feel easier." And when you're done, click on "Body Buzz" for other ways to overcome exercise roadblocks.

SAY YES TO YOGA

If most exercise options seem too hard, look into yoga. This is a gentle practice that doesn't involve a lot of sweating and hard breathing. My father was overweight most of his life. He spent his days involved in intellectual pursuits and always had a lot of things on his mind. When he turned 80, he started going to a yoga class once a week. It relaxed him, allowed him to empty his mind, and encouraged him to stretch and move in ways he was not accustomed to.

He found it a welcome change that stretched him in unexpected ways. No matter how much or how little you are used to doing, no matter how old or stiff you may feel, give it a try. Like my father, you may find it a road worth taking.

■ **Yoga is great** *for all ages, and can benefit both the body and mind.*

It takes too much time

REALLY? WE'RE TALKING ABOUT A HALF HOUR of activity each day. I bet you can waste that much time just sitting around. If you really don't think you have a half hour to spare, see if you can trade it for something else less valuable.

Simply find an alternative

Observe yourself for one day. Write down everything you do, whether it is a task, a chore, or down time. Was it all useful and productive? I doubt it. Now pick one of the nonproductive things and trade it for some exercise.

a If your chosen activities cannot be done in a half hour, try to break them into smaller pieces. Stretching for 15 minutes in the morning and taking a 15-minute walk at lunchtime adds up to the same half hour as a single bike ride.

b Combine your exercise with other activities. Remember the exercise extras? Five minutes here and 10 minutes there will quickly add up to 30. Do some gardening, walk the dog or mow the lawn. You had to do those anyway, didn't you?

c If you have a baby or toddler, see if there's a mothers' exercise group you can join. Where I live, mothers meet in the park and do exercises while their children play. The neighborhood is full of parents pushing jogging strollers at aerobic speed.

INTERNET

onhealth.webmd.com/fitness/in-depth/item/item%2C26183_1_.asp

This is a dandy article, complete with animations, that will tell you why and how to "Stretch Yourself at Work." Whether your problem is overweight or carpal tunnel syndrome, your body will thank you.

d Volunteer in your community for something that will keep you on the move instead of on the phone. Do door-to-door canvassing. Work at the local recycling center lifting bales of newspapers and dragging trash. Become a playground monitor or school-crossing guard or run errands (on foot).

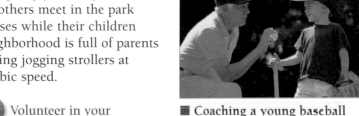

■ **Coaching a young baseball** *team can be great fun to do, and it will help keep you physically fit and active, too.*

e If you're in the office all day, do stretches at your desk. Instead of phoning, walk down the hall to see a coworker. Take your coffee break outdoors and then walk back up the stairs.

It hurts

Whoever first said, "No pain, no gain," has a lot to answer for. Safe and healthy exercise should not hurt.

Guard against getting hurt while exercising by:

a Wearing the right shoes

b Warming up, cooling down, and stretching as part of every exercise session

c Choosing exercise suited to your level of fitness and ability

d Gradually increasing weight, intensity, and speed

e Starting at a lower level if you've taken time off from your routine

f Varying your routine to give your muscles a chance to recover

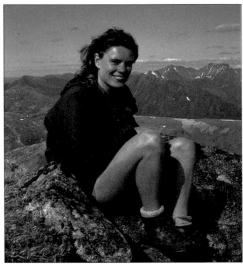

■ **Hiking is a good mix** *of brisk exercise and being out in the fresh air, but make sure your walking shoes fit well to avoid blisters.*

g Paying attention to your THR and never exercising at your MHR

h Exercising in a safe place with equipment that is in good repair

i Using good form and correct technique

j Listening to your body and stopping if something doesn't feel right

k Breathing properly: Exhale on the effort

l Drinking water to replace fluid lost through sweat

m Protecting yourself from the sun and other extremes of weather when you exercise outdoors

n Wearing protective gear as needed by the activity you choose

A **strain**, *also called a "pulled muscle" or "charley horse," occurs when a sudden movement stretches or tears muscle fibers. Pain, stiffness, and swelling result. A strain usually resolves in a few days, especially if treated with rest, ice, compression, elevation (RICE) and an anti-inflammatory pain reliever. A **sprain** is an injury to one of the ligaments that connect bone to bone. Sharp pain is usually followed by stiffness, tenderness, and swelling. Sprains are generally more serious than strains. In addition to RICE and anti-inflammatory medication, a doctor may recommend further treatment, including surgery or rehabilitative exercise.*

If you wake up the morning after feeling stiff and sore, it's a sure sign that there was something wrong with your routine the day before. Your muscles are telling you it was too fast, too heavy, too many, too far. A warm shower and some gentle stretches may help you work through the discomfort. Take a day off and do something entirely different the next day.

More serious injury

If you experience sharp pain or hear a "crack" or "pop" while lifting, pushing, pulling, or bending, stop immediately. Put an icepack on the injured area as soon as possible and seek some medical help. Pain, swelling, tenderness, and a feeling of heat at the site of the injury are signs that this is more than "too much too soon." The most common activity-related injuries are **strains** and **sprains**. They may sound the same, but a strain is a muscle injury and a sprain is an injury affecting joints and connective tissue.

If you become injured while exercising, do not try to diagnose the problem yourself. Do not ask a friend or someone at your gym.

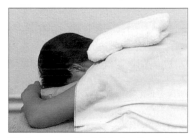

There's enough myth and misinformation about sports injuries to fill a fat book. This is no time for amateur hour. Instead, call a medical professional. Describe the problem and the circumstances. You may be advised to come in to be examined or even to go to a hospital emergency room. Or you may be told it's safe to wait two or three days to see if the pain and swelling subside. In the meantime, you will do yourself no further harm, and may even help, by giving yourself the RICE treatment: rest, ice, compression, elevation

1 Rest the injured part of your body. Stop what you're doing and do not resume activity until the condition has resolved.

2 Apply ice or a chilled gel-pack to the injured part. Cover the icebag or pack with a washcloth or towel so it does not contact your skin directly. Leave it on for no more than 10 minutes at a time, then take it off for 10 minutes, and keep repeating the cycle. This will prevent you from giving yourself frostbite.

■ **A covered, chilled** *gel-pack placed on your injured muscle will reduce pain and inflammation.*

3 If possible, wrap the injured part in an elastic compression bandage to give it support and help reduce swelling. You may wish to continue wearing the bandage or an elasticized brace for a while to protect the injured part.

4 Elevate the injured part with a pillow or a stack of books.

In addition, you may get relief from an anti-inflammatory pain reliever such as aspirin or ibuprofen, which will also help reduce swelling.

Check your technique

As soon as you are feeling better, get advice from a trainer, instructor, or other knowledgeable person to avoid injury again. It may be a matter of using lighter weights, or bending your knees, or changing your technique slightly.

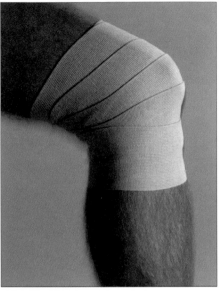

■ **Knee injuries can** *be very painful. Strapping your knee in an elastic bandage will aid the healing process and may help you continue to play your normal sport.*

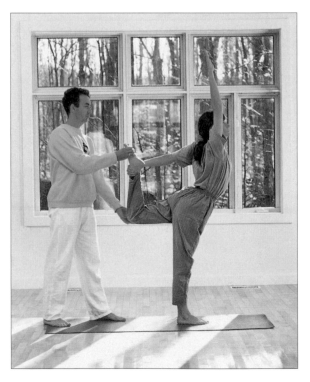

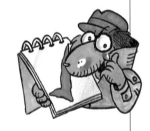

Have the trainer watch you for a while and talk you through the activity you are doing.

Review your warm-up, cool-down, and stretching techniques. If you are in a class that does not allow for enough of this, schedule some time on your own before and after the class. This may be a good time to have a lesson or to do a session or two with a personal trainer.

■ **Ask your trainer** *to show you the correct form, posture, and technique, or alternative moves that will not stress the part you have injured.*

I've been sick

DO YOU REALLY HAVE TO STOP EXERCISING *if you're feeling under the weather? It depends on two factors: how sick you are and what activity you are doing.*

If you have a cold, seasonal allergies, or menstrual cramps, don't let these serve as an excuse. Exercise won't make these conditions worse, and in some cases, they might even make them better.

Exercise stimulates the release of adrenaline, the hormone also known as epinephrine. Among its useful roles, this hormone is a natural decongestant.

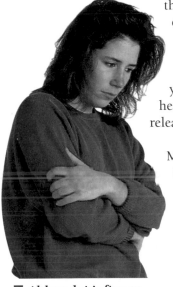

Unlike the kind that comes in pill form, adrenaline does not make you feel jittery. It makes you feel supercharged. And the nice thing about *endogenous* epinephrine is that the dose is adjusted by your own body. It's like a custom-made time-release capsule: You move your muscles and get your heart pumping, and just the right amount of the "drug" is released into your bloodstream.

Menstrual cramps may also be relieved by exercise. Increased blood flow to the muscles can lessen cramps. Exercise also stimulates endorphins, the natural painkillers that have an affinity for the same brain receptors as opium.

All in all, it sounds like exercise is the best medicine for minor physical ills. You may want to lower the intensity of your workout and pay closer attention to how you are feeling, but there's really no reason to stop.

If you have flu symptoms – fever, headache, body aches – or if you are vomiting, have diarrhea, or have severe chest congestion with a bad cough, it makes sense to stop exercising until these symptoms pass.

DEFINITION

Endogenous means "coming from within." That is, something that the body makes rather than taking it in from an outside source (exogenous). Cholesterol is another example of a substance that can be both endogenous and exogenous. The cholesterol made by your liver is endogenous; dietary cholesterol contained in food you eat is exogenous.

■ **Although it's fine to exercise** *if you are suffering from a minor ailment, you should stop if you have a temperature or if you are feeling seriously unwell.*

It's simply too expensive

FOR EVERY $1,000-A-YEAR HEALTH CLUB, *there is a $19.95-a-month gym. For every $100-a-round green's fee, there is a community softball program. If signing up for a semester's worth of classes costs a lump sum you can't manage, find a pay-as-you-go alternative. Don't let the price get in the way of the prize. Many activities require little or no special equipment, club membership, or lessons.*

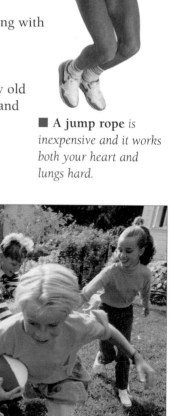

a Try jumping rope, dancing in your living room, sparring with a partner, flying a kite.

b You can ride a bike that has fewer than 20 speeds and doesn't boast a titanium frame; there's probably a rusty old one in your garage that needs no more than some oil and a new seat.

■ **A jump rope** *is inexpensive and it works both your heart and lungs hard.*

c Can't afford a stairclimber? Just find some stairs and climb them instead.

d Running is free, and so is playing tag with your children in the backyard.

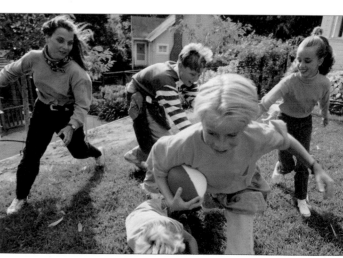

■ **Playing tag with your** *children in the backyard will give you the opportunity to spend more time with them, and can be your exercise session for the day.*

_e_ Exercise videos are inexpensive, and you can swap them with friends, or tape a series from a cable exercise program.

_f_ Personal trainers may be an extravagance, but there are dozens of web sites that offer personalized programs with a few clicks of the mouse.

The perfect gift

If money really is an issue, make it a wish or a special gift you give yourself. Instead of a new outfit or a restaurant meal, ask for a few classes, a new pair of running shoes, or membership at the Y. Make it a reward for losing 10 pounds or a graduation present when you reach one of your milestones.

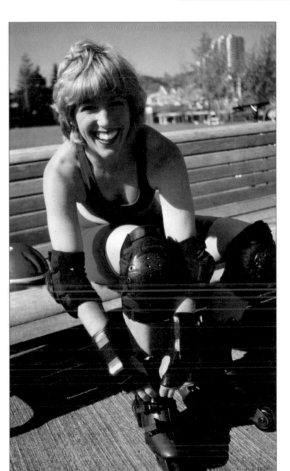

Make the investment worth it. Sometimes spending money works as a motivator. If the price of membership is what keeps you going to the gym, it's money well spent. If you'll really use those inline skates now that you've invested in a new set of wheels and safety equipment, you're on a roll.

Whatever it costs you, regular exercise is worth it.

You may well save money in the long run by avoiding the cost of medical care and time off from work for weight-related illnesses. Being active is a matter of health, not wealth.

■ **You deserve regular treats** _when you achieve another weight-loss goal. If you have always wanted to go inline skating, buy yourself a pair of skates and go out and enjoy yourself._

I'll be away from home

ONE OF THE LAMEST EXCUSES *for dropping an exercise program is being on the road. Whether work or vacation takes you away from your local gym or exercise class or simply makes you change your routine, that's no reason to break your stride.*

Business trips

If you use being away on business as an excuse for shelving your daily exercise routine, I've got news for you. There isn't a hotel, motel, or conference center in this country, and probably not anywhere else in the world, that doesn't have a health club or at least a swimming pool available for guests. In all likelihood, you'll be able to continue your routine, possibly even in surroundings far more sophisiticated than the ones you have at home.

Many gyms and exercise clubs are part of national chains or federations that give visiting privileges to members from out of town.

If you belong to a club, check out whether there is one where you're visiting before you hit the road. You may have a home away from home without even knowing it.

If for some reason that is not practical or possible, there will be a television in your room. Instead of watching the pay-per-view movie while lying on the bed and munching from the minibar, find a televised exercise class and join in.

Whatever you do, never leave for a business trip without packing a swimsuit, a workout outfit, and a comfortable pair of sneakers or running shoes.

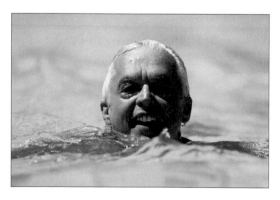

If you think the facilities will be limited, bring along an exercise video in case there's a VCR, or a jump rope and a pair of weights. Being unequipped is not an excuse; it's just poor planning.

■ **Most hotel or motels** *have swimming pools, so there is no excuse to miss out on your daily laps when you're away from home on business.*

Vacations

You have a lot more control over where you go and what you do when you're on the road for vacation. Plan a holiday that's action packed. That need not limit you to skiing in the Alps and scuba diving in the Caribbean. Consider the following:

a. Do you want to go on a cruise? You'll find onboard pools, gyms, and exercise classes, not to mention dancing long into the night.

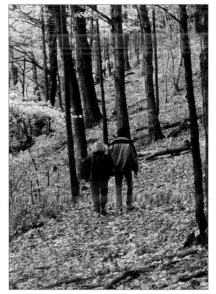

b. Are you touring a foreign land? Walking is a major activity for tourists, from Australia to Zanzibar. You can walk in cities and in the countryside, visiting museums, antiquities, or natural attractions. Do as the natives do, whether it's strolling in a park or dancing in a public square. There are many biking and walking tours, geared to all interests, ages, and levels of skill. Think about signing up for one.

■ **A road trip** *does not mean you have to sit in the car all day. Plan regular stops, get out, and go for walks.*

c. Will you spend a week at a beach resort? Instead of lying on a blanket, pack paddles and balls, a Frisbee™, a kite, and any other items that will keep you vertical and moving around.

d. Driving across country with family? Choose overnight stops with swimming pools and do some laps to work out the kinks. Stop frequently to stretch your legs, climb a hill to get a good view, walk around a historic site, or climb a historic monument. Think about national parks and other outdoor attractions. Explore the towns where you stop. Find the local golf course, bowling alley, or dance hall.

e. Visiting relatives? Let them know you want some action. They may be able to get guest passes at a local gym, sign you up for lessons or classes, find out about running or other sports events in the area. Unless you let your hosts know you're in an active frame of mind, you'll end up sitting around.

You may not be able to follow your usual routine while you're away from home, but there's plenty you can do to ensure that you return from your holidays looking fitter, not fatter.

INTERNET

www.teleport.com /~walking/hiking.html

The Walking & Hiking Homepage is a treasure trove of information and links to treks, tours, clubs, and places to travel on foot in the United States and throughout the world.

It doesn't seem to be working

YOU'VE BEEN EXERCISING FAITHFULLY, but you're not seeing a dramatic weight loss. Right about now you're asking yourself, "What's the point?"

You may be using the wrong yardstick to measure your success. Rather than looking at the scale, cast an eye on how you look and feel.

Back in Chapter 1, you examined yourself in the mirror and noted all the parts of your body you wished were otherwise. When was the last time you took such a hard look? Have you noticed that your tummy is trimmer? That your arms jiggle less and your thighs are firmer? There's a good chance that you've replaced fat with muscle without even knowing it. And because muscle tissue weighs more than fat, you've gained strength rather than losing weight.

Even more important is how you feel. When was the last time you took a fitness test? Take another one now and write the results in your personal database. Are there improvements in your strength, flexibility, and endurance? Does it take longer for you to reach your THR and less time to return to you RHR? These are all signs that increased activity is really paying fitness dividends.

What about your mood and self-image? Do you feel more able? More in command? Are there things you do regularly you never thought you'd do? Do you have more "get up and go"? Are you more involved in positive pursuits? Do you have more energy?

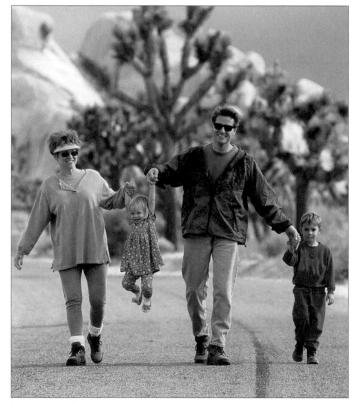

■ **Don't get upset** *if your exercise routine is not bringing the weight-loss results you'd hoped for. Just appreciate the extra stamina and energy you have for family activities.*

I'd be very surprised if the answer isn't "Yes!" Being more active isn't a temporary solution. It's a lifestyle choice. Keeping it up will keep you younger and healthier all the days of your life.

A simple summary

✔ Don't use boredom as an excuse to be inactive. There's a wide range of pursuits to suit every temperament. It's simply a matter of finding a few that turn you on.

✔ Choose activities that fit your skill level and work your way up as you become more fit. If it's too hard, lower the intensity or frequency, or try something else.

✔ If exercise takes too big a chunk out of your day, do it in smaller bites or combine it with other things you do.

✔ Being active shouldn't hurt. If it does, check your technique and your equipment. Be sure to warm up, cool down, and stretch.

✔ Feeling under the weather is not necessarily a reason to sit on the bench. In many cases, staying active will actually make you feel better. Ask your doctor if you're in doubt.

✔ Exercise does not have to equal expense. There are many low- or no-cost choices to explore. If you still think it's too expensive, consider this: So is the price of illness and disability you risk by being sedentary.

✔ Don't take a time-out from your exercise routine when you travel for business or pleasure. Make every trip an active one, and don't forget to pack your weight-loss notebook. You may even come home slimmer than when you left.

✔ Measure the success of your more active lifestyle in terms of fitness, energy, and vitality, not weight loss alone.

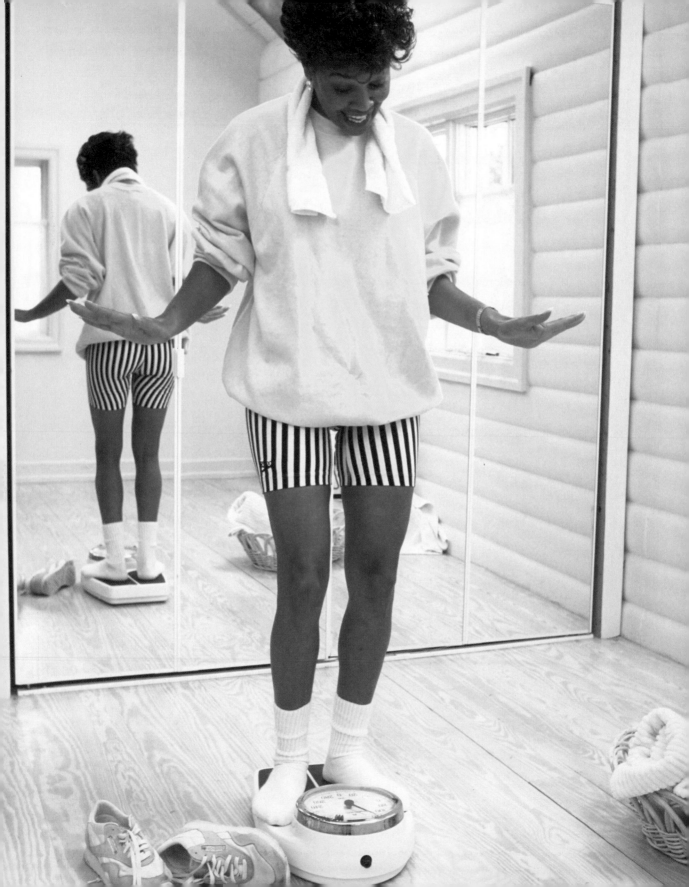

Chapter 20

You've Done It

YOU'RE A NEW PERSON: You're fit, you have good eating and exercise habits, you look good and feel great. Even if you haven't achieved all of your goals, you've come a long way from Chapter 1. But this is not the end of the road. In many ways, it's a new beginning. Maintaining a healthy weight and staying fit is a process. Whatever you do, don't give up. Build on your success.

In this chapter...

✓ A new you

✓ The name of the game is maintain

✓ Evaluate

✓ Take it to the next level

✓ Lifetime eating

✓ As you grow older

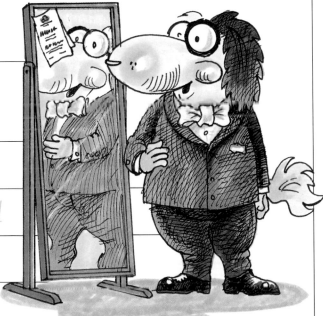

LOSING WEIGHT IS A GREAT ACHIEVEMENT: CELEBRATE THE NEW YOU AND AN EXCITING NEW BEGINNING

A new you

LOSING WEIGHT IS NOT A HOBBY *and being fit is not a passing fad. They are a way of life. Read this chapter once a month to remind yourself why and how to keep up your good habits and keep track of your progress.*

Begin by taking a thorough inventory of the new you. Take out your weight-loss notebook and turn to the personal database. If you like, mark a new column "The new me." Put in today's date and take your measurements in all of the categories.

Now make some lists. Begin with "I'm so proud," a list of your accomplishments. The second list should be called something like "There's still work to do." Write down the areas that have not improved, or not improved as much as you hope. The third list should be called "Major hurdles." This is for the intractable problems, things you can't seem to change and may have to live with.

Don't write off the things you can't seem to change as lost causes.

Seeing how much you have accomplished may give you the self-confidence you need to tackle these toughies. They may be good candidates for new long-term goals. They may be easier to conquer now that you are fitter. Or, to tell the truth, your goals may be unrealistic. Spot-reducing, becoming an Olympic athlete, and washboard abs at the age of 70 may simply not be in the cards.

Renew your contract

Pull out the contract you signed way back when and reread it. Have you fulfilled the terms? A good contract is renewable, though sometimes it needs revision. Make whatever changes are appropriate and draw up a rider including all the new provisions. Sign it, date it, and get a witness. You may want to frame the first contract to show off what you accomplished, or even make yourself a certificate of completion and hang it on your mirror or refrigerator.

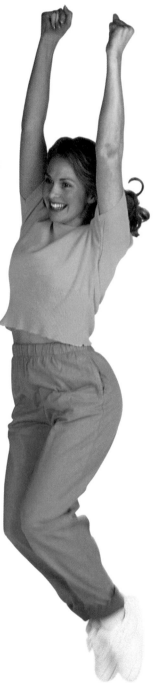

■ **Success feels great,** *and you have reason to be proud. Just keep up the good work.*

My personal database

Date	10/1	12/1	3/1	6/1
My weight	200 lbs	176 lbs	166 lbs	159 lbs
My height	5 ft 4in →→→			
My BMI (body mass index)	34.3	30.2	28.5	27.3
My ideal weight range	107–147 →→→			
Number of pounds more than ideal weight	53 lbs	29 lbs	19 lbs	12 lbs

MY BODY TYPE

	10/1	12/1	3/1	6/1
Waist size	40 in	35 in	34 in	33 in
Hip size	46 in	43 in	42 in	41 in
My waist-to-hip ratio (WHR)	0.86	0.81	0.80	0.80

I am an apple or (pear) (circle one)

My main body type problem is: (circle one)

I am at higher risk for diabetes, high blood pressure, heart disease

(Losing weight and keeping it off may be harder for me)

MY MEASUREMENTS

	10/1	12/1	3/1	6/1
Chest/bust	38 in	36 in	35 in	35 in
Upper thigh	21 in	20 in	19 in	19 in
Calf	14 in	14 in	13½ in	13½ in
Upper arm	14 in	13 in	12½ in	12½ in
Lower arm	10 in	9½ in	9 in	9 in
Other				

■ **Comparing your current measurements** *with your previous ones will show you at a glance how much you have achieved on your weight-loss program and where improvements can still be made.*

The name of the game is maintain

I WAS HOPING not to have to mention this, but you do need to know that maintaining weight loss is even more difficult than losing weight to begin with. A staggering percentage of people who lose weight through diet gain all or most of it back within a very short time. Some give up and some start playing with the diet yo-yo. Losing weight but not maintaining the loss is horribly discouraging, and all too common.

The simple truth is that dieting alone does not work. Making wise food choices is only part of the answer; leading an active lifestyle is the key.

Regular exercise – to keep your metabolism burning, your muscles strong and toned, and your heart and lungs working efficiently – is crucial to maintaining a healthy weight.

Keep monitoring

Over the past months, you've been keeping your weight-loss journal, writing down what you eat and how much you exercise, and periodically taking a yardstick and measuring tape to your life and body. You may be tired of this routine or it may have become a matter of easy habit.

Don't abandon your weight-loss journal. You may be able to do it less often, but don't discard it altogether.

Keeping a weight-loss journal has already helped you track your progress. No matter how far you still have to go, it will continue to be an important tool. It will serve to motivate you as well as give you an early warning signal if you start to slip.

It's a good idea to maintain an awareness of your weight. Decide how often you want to weigh-in and whether you also want to keep measuring key parts of your body. Weekly may be too often, but monthly or quarterly are reasonable. You will probably see less dramatic changes, but be sure to act fast if you notice any slippage. If you have gained a pound, it's not a cause for panic, but it is a cause for caution. A gain of more than 2 percent of your current body weight should set off an alarm.

If, for example, you now weigh 150 pounds, a 3-pound gain is a danger signal. Try to figure out what has caused it. Have you added more fat to your diet? Are you snacking more? Have some foods crept off your blacklist and onto your daily menu? Are you exercising less or less vigorously?

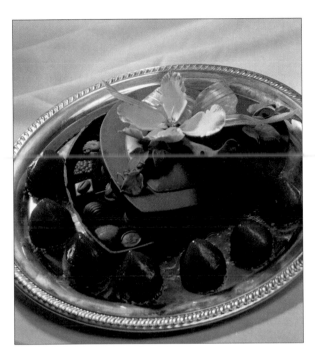

It is far easier to lose 3 newly gained pounds than to start all over again at square one.

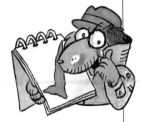

■ **Were you given chocolates** *you simply could not resist? If you can pinpoint the culprit for your weight gain, kick it in the butt. If you cannot, reinstate your daily food and activity diaries for at least a week.*

FACTS ABOUT FADS

There may soon be hard scientific evidence about the most effective and healthiest weight-loss diet. In a field filled with controversy, not to mention more diets than you can go on in a lifetime, the USDA is stepping in with controlled studies of the two ends of the spectrum: the high-fat, low-carbohydrate regimen espoused by Robert Atkins and others versus the low-fat, high-carbohydrate approach of Dean Ornish. Preliminary results are expected sometime in 2001.

In the meantime, Secretary of Health and Human Services Donna Shalala has this to say: "When it comes to crash diets and fad diets, the guidelines are clear: Stop doing them. They won't last. Instead, take the weight off slowly and steadily through a powerful combination of sensible eating and physical activity."

But you knew that already.

Evaluate

EVEN IF YOU ARE SUCCESSFUL *at maintaining your weight or continuing to lose, if that is your aim, it's worthwhile to periodically evaluate what you are doing. Ask yourself what's working and whether these strategies have become comfortable habits or feel like burdens. If they are burdensome, can you replace them with others that will be equally effective but fit better into your life? Take a look at what does not seem to be working. These strategies should be substituted for other, more effective strategies.*

The best source for this analysis is your journal. Are you still a slave to old habits? Have your triggers changed or do the same moods, people, and circumstances throw you back into lazing about and eating irresponsibly? If your evaluation reveals that you are slacking off on activity, read this as a red alert. Now is not the time to slow down. Reducing your activity level is a slippery slope, and you may soon find yourself back on the couch with a bag of chips.

Simple stamina

No truer words were spoken than "Use it or lose it." One of the first things to go when you stop exercising is stamina. Studies have shown that measures of endurance drop as early as 3 weeks after a person stops exercising. Muscle strength and bulk start to wane in about 4 weeks and soon reach their old flabby state. Weight gain is rapid, due to the double whammy of lower energy need and slower metabolism. The last thing you want to do after all your hard work is to find yourself back at square one.

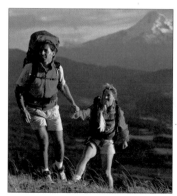

■ **You may have come** *a long way, but you did it one step at a time.*

Motivation update

If you need to put a new spark into your plan, one of the best things you can do is to update your motivators. Look back at what got you going in the first place. Do these dreams still turn you on? If your closet is now filled with clothes that you like and your social life makes you happy, what else might you reach for? If your doctor gave you a clean bill of health at your last checkup, is it time to try some more ambitious physical pursuits?

Take a look at the milestones you originally set for yourself. Have you reached them all? If not, make a new list of those that remain and add some new ones. As always, arrange them in small steps toward a farther goal.

Take it to the next level

ONE OF THE MOST GRATIFYING THINGS *about a successful plan is the strength it gives you to do more. When you started this campaign, your exercise options were probably quite limited. As an overweight person with a sedentary lifestyle, your skills and abilities were low. Walking, stretching, strength training with light weights, and beginning exercise classes were a good place to start. Now you are ready to rev it up.*

Reassess your fitness

Before you think about revving it up, take the activity/fitness self-test again. You can do the one in Chapter 8 or try one of the online self-assessment tests. If you do the test in this book, be sure to update your personal database in the same way as you did for your weight and measurements so you can see the improvement clearly.

INTERNET

www.onhealth.com /fitness/in-depth/item /item,35662_1_1.asp

Here's another fitness assessment test, and a good one too.

MY FITNESS FACTS

	2	6	7	8
Lifestyle/activity score	2	6	7	8
Endurance				
Number of jumping jacks	15	20	30	40
Pulse	180	176	170	160
Time to RHR	3 mins	3 mins	2 ½ mins	2 mins
Strength				
Number of chest lifts	10	20	30	50
Flexibility				
Inches reached	25	27	29	30

■ **Compare your current levels of fitness** *with your previous ones by dating and filling in the new figures in your personal database. Do these show an increase in fitness?*

If the facts reveal a fitter you, it's time to challenge yourself. The simplest thing is to do more of the same, but do it longer, harder, and faster. More interesting is to move to a more complex level. Consider the following changes:

a If you have been exercising at home alone, are you ready to join a gym?

b If you have been stretching, are you ready for a 45-minute workout class?

c If you have been taking all-purpose calisthenics classes, how about kick boxing or tae bo?

d If you've been swimming laps, why not do it for time rather than distance?

e If you have been running, are you ready for a minimarathon?

f If you've done your time on a stationary bike, jump on the kind that moves and go conquer some hills.

g If you've been trudging on the treadmill, try some interval training by breaking into a run for one minute out of every five.

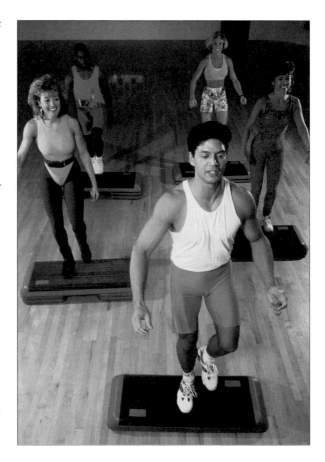

The idea is to stick with the kinds of things you like to do, but do them more vigorously. Another approach is to work on a new part of your body or a different aspect of fitness. If your arms are strong but your abs are still flabby, focus on exercise that will strengthen your abdominal muscles. Your back will benefit too. If you've been concentrating on becoming more flexible, add cardiorespiratory fitness to your workout.

■ **If you have been doing aerobics**, *think about moving up a level by trying salsa aerobics, or jazzercise, or getting up on those steps.*

Lifetime eating

IS IT TIME TO "GO OFF" YOUR DIET YET? *No, not if it means going back to eating like a fat person. Yes, if it means adjusting the restrictions to the new realities.*

Even after you've reached your ideal weight, calories still count and they always will. The principle of calories in–calories out still holds.

The number of calories you need for basal metabolism and to maintain your weight has changed if your weight has changed. Figure out your new daily calorie needs based on your current weight. If you don't remember how to do it, look back at Chapter 5. Don't forget to add your lifestyle percentage. This is where you will see the real payoff.

Your baseline calorie needs may have decreased as your weight has, but you've lost that weight by increasing activity. That means you need more calories to fuel all that extra activity.

My basal metabolic rate (BMR)	2,000	1,760	1,660	1,590
My daily calorie needs to maintain weight	2,400	2,288	2,158	2,067
My daily calorie goal to lose weight	1,900	1,788	1,658	1,567

■ **As you lose weight** *record your new BMR details and calorie needs in your personal database so that you know what you're aiming for.*

If you still want to lose more, you'll have to restrict calories to a level below your daily calorie needs. You decide how much weight you want to lose and how quickly you want to do it. By now you should know the math by heart: 3,500 calories = 1 pound.

If you are happy with your weight and want to maintain it, you can begin to relax your intake restrictions. Don't go nuts! Especially if they're drenched with hot fudge atop a banana split. You may be relaxing your restrictions, but don't relax your vigilance. And whatever you do, don't stop being active. If you do, you'll lose the benefit of the lifestyle percentage and start gaining pounds.

Be vigilant

This is a good time to ask yourself again what food means to you. Take the food behavior test in Chapter 7 again. Many of your answers will be different, but some might be the same. Grade yourself, highlighting food behaviors you think will still cause problems. It would also be a good idea to reinstate the practices of the early days of your diet.

1. Make menus: Plan what you will eat and deliberately build in the extras. Count the calories you are adding and make them count. An extra 100 calories that will not give you pleasure or feel like a treat is 100 calories wasted.

2. Keep your diary, recording everything you eat. Compare it to the menus and make a note if you go over your limit.

3. Make notes of your moods, triggers, and any other observations that will help you keep track of how well you are adjusting.

At the first sign that things are getting out of hand, stop, go back a few steps, and get back in control.

Everybody is different. You may be like a recovering alcoholic or other substance abuser. It may be impossible for you to have even a little of something previously forbidden. On the other hand, you may have conquered your addictions and no longer eat compulsively or impulsively. It may be possible for you to have a little.

As you grow older

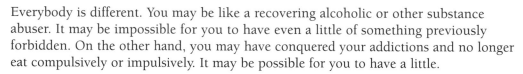

MOST PEOPLE GAIN WEIGHT *as they grow older, typically adding 5 to 10 pounds per decade. That does not mean this is normal or even natural. To the contrary, the facts of normal aging suggest that weight should be lost, not gained, since there is a progressive loss of the two heaviest body tissues: muscle and bone. So what's going on? The answer can be found in the principle of calories in–calories out.*

BMR and calorie needs decrease with age. So does activity level. You can't do much to change the first two facts, but you can do a lot about the third.

It is a myth that we have less energy for active pursuits as we grow older. For too many of us, it's a self-fulfilling prophecy. The less we do, the less we feel like doing.

We lose the mood-enhancing benefits of activity as quickly as we lose muscle tone and cardiorespiratory fitness. These combine to make us lose our independence as well.

If you are still young and vigorous, now is the time to invest in a healthy old age. If you are in middle age, think of it as prime time. If you are already on the far side of 65, it's not too late.

Change your eating habits

My teenage son can polish off a quart of milk, two bananas, and a box of raisins in one sitting. He packs in calories like there's no tomorrow and seems only to grow taller, not wider. My middle-aged brothers, former string beans both, have gradually turned to apples. The problem is they never changed their eating habits, but they are much less active than they were as young men. It's simply a fact that we need less food after our growing years.

The biggest drop in calorie requirements occurs after age 20, when calorie needs decrease by about 20 percent. It levels off for a few decades and then drops about 10 percent at age 50. At age 75, there is another 10 percent reduction.

Keep these watersheds in mind as you grow older and adjust the way you eat accordingly. Keep one eye on the scale and the other on your calorie counter.

Keep active

Leave the rocking chair on the front porch and keep moving. You may have to eat less, but there's no reason to reduce the amount of time you spend on exercise. When you engage in aerobic activity, pay attention to your heartbeat. Remember, your MHR lowers with age, so your THR does too. MHR is 220 minus your age; your target zone is between 60 and 80 percent of that.

Look at the chart in Chapter 8 and find your target zone. This will change every 5 years, so keep your exercise intensity up to date. You may change the sorts of activities you do, but even that may not be necessary. It goes without saying that you should check with your doctor before embarking on a more active routine if you are over 65, especially if you have been relatively inactive before. The chances are good you'll get a medical blessing, though it may come with some tips on exercising safely.

Trivia...

According to the National Institute on Aging, regular exercise is more popular among seniors than it is in the generation just below them. Around 32 percent of Americans age 65 and older say they have, and follow, an exercise plan, whereas only 30 percent of those aged 45 to 64 do so. It's still not enough in either age group!

INTERNET

www.phys.com/self/eat

"Eat for Your Life" details healthy eating strategies for your 20s, 30s, and 40s.

Fitness facts

- Weight-bearing exercise delays the bone loss of osteoporosis

- Aerobic exercise maintains a healthy cardiovascular system

- Resistance training delays and possibly even prevents loss of muscle mass and strength

- Stretching exercise improves flexibility and balance

- Being active promotes mental alertness

INTERNET

www.thriveonline.com /health/srhealth.html

Want some more ideas? Check out this 50+ health page at Thrive Online.

You can do it at any age

If you can bear another family story, I'll tell you one about my mother. The summer she was 80 she injured her knee during her regular weekly tennis game. She had been playing tennis for years and, prior to the injury, saw no reason to stop. She had the knee X-rayed and when she went in to see the doctor, he picked up the film, frowned, and muttered something about having been given the wrong file. "This is the knee of a 40-year-old woman," he insisted. In fact, it was my mother's knee, its bones as dense as a person's half her age.

Here's a baker's dozen of activities for which age is no bar:

1. Bicycling, stationary and otherwise

2. Bowling

3. Dancing

4. Golf

5. Housework, including vacuuming, dusting, washing windows

6. Light weight training: free weights or training apparatus

7. Ping pong

8. Stretching

9. Swimming

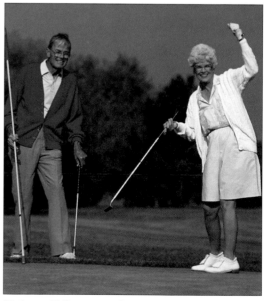

■ **Overall fitness** *makes it possible to remain active and independent well into old age.*

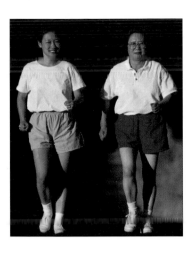

10 T'ai chi

11 Walking

12 Yardwork, including gardening, lawn mowing, and raking leaves

13 Yoga

■ **Maintain your fitness** *as you grow older by making active walking part of your everyday routine.*

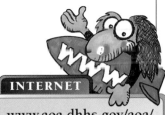

INTERNET

www.aoa.dhhs.gov/aoa/ pages/agepages/ exercise.html

"Feeling Fit for Life" is an online brochure from the Administration on Aging.

A simple summary

✓ Update your personal database with your current measurements to celebrate the changes you have made.

✓ Focus on maintenance: Make sure you keep the weight off and the activity on.

✓ Continue to monitor your weight and your exercise plan – don't be tempted to discard your weight-loss journal.

✓ Act fast if you find yourself sliding back into old habits: Revive your food and activity diaries and zero in on the problem.

✓ Evaluate what works and what does not. Your body is a work in progress, so don't hesitate to make modifications.

✓ Challenge yourself and use your new vitality and new skills.

✓ Carefully and gradually make the transition from eating for weight loss to eating for life.

✓ Make adjustments to your calorie intake as you grow older and your needs change.

✓ Keep your commitment to an active lifestyle. It will pay off as you grow older.

My personal database

Date				
My weight				
My height	→			
My BMI (body mass index)				
My ideal weight range	→			
Number of pounds more than ideal weight				

MY BODY TYPE

Waist size				
Hip size				
My waist-to-hip ratio (WHR)				

I am an apple or pear (circle one)

My main body type problem is: (circle one)

    I am at higher risk for diabetes, high blood pressure, heart disease

    Losing weight and keeping it off may be harder for me

MY MEASUREMENTS

Chest/bust				
Upper thigh				
Calf				
Upper arm				
Lower arm				
Other				

Date				
My resting heart rate (RHR)				
My maximum heart rate (MHR)				
My target heart rate (THR) 60%/80%				
My basal metabolic rate (BMR)				
My daily calorie needs to maintain weight				
My daily calorie goal to lose weight				

MY FITNESS FACTS

Lifestyle/activity score				
Endurance:				
Number of jumping jacks				
Pulse				
Time to RHR				
Strength:				
Number of chest lifts				
Flexibility:				
Inches reached				

NOTES

Weight-loss timetable

MY LONG-TERM GOALS

MY MILESTONES

	Date	Goal weight	Comment
1			
2			
3			
4			
5			
6			
7			
8			
9			
10			
11			
12			

PHOTOCOPY THIS PAGE FOR YOUR OWN USE

Daily food diary

Day   Date

BREAKFAST *Time*

FOOD	SERVINGS	CALORIES

COMMENTS *(hunger level, place, people, etc.)*

LUNCH *Time*

FOOD	SERVINGS	CALORIES

COMMENTS *(hunger level, place, people, etc.)*

Daily food diary

Day _____ Date _____

DINNER Time _____

FOOD	SERVINGS	CALORIES

COMMENTS (hunger level, place, people, etc.)

SNACKS

TIME	FOOD	SERVINGS	CALORIES

COMMENTS (hunger level, place, people, etc.)

Water: (Check each 8 oz. glass) ○   ○   ○   ○   ○   ○   ○   ○

Total calories: _____

Activity timetable

MY LONG-TERM GOALS

MY MILESTONES

	Date	Activity goal	Comment
1			
2			
3			
4			
5			
6			
7			
8			
9			
10			
11			
12			

Daily activity diary

Day   Date

Activity	Time	Duration	Calories burned	Place	Comments (mood, place, people, etc.)

NOTES

Day   Date

Activity	Time	Duration	Calories burned	Place	Comments (mood, place, people, etc.)

NOTES

Daily activity diary

Day _____ Date _____

Activity	Time	Duration	Calories burned	Place	Comments (mood, place, people, etc.)

NOTES

Day _____ Date _____

Activity	Time	Duration	Calories burned	Place	Comments (mood, place, people, etc.)

NOTES

Other resources

Books

The American Dietetic Association Complete Food & Nutrition Guide
Roberta Larson Duyff, John Wiley, 1998.

The American Yoga Association Beginner's Manual
Alice Christensen, Fireside, 1987.

The Beginning Runner's Handbook: The Proven 13-week Walk Run Program
Ian MacNeill and Sports Medicine Council, Greystone Publishing, 1999.

Fat is a Feminist Issue: A Self Help Guide for Compulsive Eaters
Susie Orbach, Berkley Publishing Group, 1991.

Fitting in Fitness: Hundreds of Simple Ways to Put More Physical Activity into Your Life
American Heart Association, Times Books, 1997.

365 Ways to Get Out the Fat: A Tip a Day to Trim the Fat Away
American Heart Association, Times Books, 1998.

Newsletters and pamphlets

Mayo Clinic Health Letter
Subscription Services
P.O. Box 53889
Boulder, CO 80322
800-333-9037

Nutrition Action Health Letter
Center for Science in the Public Interest (CSPI)
1875 Connecticut Ave NW, Suite 300
Washington, DC 20009
202-332-9110

Tufts University Health & Nutrition Letter
P.O. Box 57843
Boulder, CO 80321
800-274-7581
www.healthletter.tufts.edu

University of California, Berkeley Wellness Letter
Health Letter Associates
P.O. Box 420-235
Palm Coast, FL 32142
800-829-9080

Easy Food Tips for Heart Healthy Eating (1996)
AHA Diet, An Eating Plan for Healthy Americans (1996)
Nutritious Nibbles: A Guide to Healthy Snacking (1996)
All available from the American Heart Association (see opposite).

Associations

American Council on Exercise
5820 Oberlin Drive
Suite 102
San Diego, CA 92121
858-535-8227
www.acefitness.org

American Diabetes Association
Customer Service
1701 North Beauregard Street
Alexandria, VA 22311
800-DIABETES (800-342-2383)
www.diabetes.org

American Dietetic Association
216 W. Jackson Blvd
Chicago, IL 60606
800-877-1600
Consumer Nutrition Hotline:
800-366-1655
www.eatright.org

American Heart Association
National Center
7272 Greenville Avenue
Dallas, TX 75231
800-AHA-USA1
www.americanheart.org
Nutrition website:
www.deliciousdecisions.org

American Medical Association
515 North State Street
Chicago, IL 60610
312-464-5000
www.ama-assn.org/consumer.htm

International Food Information Council Foundation
1100 Connecticut Avenue NW, Suite 430
Washington, DC 20036
202-296-6450
ificinfo.health.org

National Council Against Health Fraud, Inc.
P.O. Box 1276
Loma Linda, CA 92354
909-824-4690
www.ncahf.org

Government agencies

Department of Agriculture:
Food and Nutrition Information Center
National Agricultural Library
Room 304
10301 Baltimore Avenue
Beltsville, MD 20705
301-504-5719
www.nal.usda.gov/fnic

Department of Agriculture:
Nutrient Data Laboratory
USDA Agricultural Research Service
Beltsville Human Nutrition Research
Center 4700 River Rd
Unit 89
Riverdale, MD 20737
301-734-8491
www.nal.usda.gov/fnic/foodcomp/

Department of Agriculture:
Center for Nutrition Policy and Promotion
1120 20th Street NW
Suite 200, North Lobby
Washington DC 20036
202-418-2312
www.usda.gov/fcs/cnpp.htm

Department of Health and Human Services
Consumer Information Center
Department WW
P.O. Box 100
Pueblo, CO 81009
www.pueblo.gsa.gov/food.htm

Food and Drug Administration (FDA)
Center for Food Safety and Applied
Nutrition Food Labeling
5600 Fishers Lane (HFE-88)
Room 1685
Rockville, MD 20847
301-443-9767
vm.cfsan.fda.gov/label.html

National Heart, Lung, and Blood Institute (NHLBI)
Information Center
P.O. Box 30105
Bethesda, MD 20824
301-251-1222
www.nhlbi.nih.gov/health/pubs

National Institute of Diabetes and Digestive and
Kidney Diseases (NIDDK)
Weight-control Information Network
1 WIN Way
Bethesda, MD 20892
800-WIN-8098
www.niddk.nih.gov/health/nutrit/nutrit.htm

Support

Overeaters Anonymous
World Service Office (WSO)
6075 Zenith Court NE
Rio Rancho
NM 87124
505-891-2664
www.overeatersanonymous.org

Take Off Pounds Sensibly (TOPS®)
4575 South Fifth Street
Milwaukee
WI 53207
800-932-8677
www.tops.org

Web sites

Diet and nutrition

www.about.com/health/weightloss

"Doubtful Diets" will help you steer clear of what doesn't work or might harm you.

www.caloriecontrol.org

The Calorie Control Council offers information and ideas on cutting calories, plus links to other reliable sources of information.

www.calorieking.com

Check out this web site for healthy low-fat recipes.

www.cyberdiet.com

You'll learn how to cut the fat and calories from your favorite foods with the "Recipe Makeover" in the "Diet & Nutrition" section. Click on "Dining Out" for tips on finding "lite" dining choices; organized by cuisine and food type.

www.diabetes.org

A good place to find ideas for low-cal recipes and other tips for healthy eating, whether you have diabetes or not.

www.4weightloss.com

Look here for links to several magazines where you'll find lots of weight-wise cooking advice.

www.hcrc.org/faqs/atkins.html

Healthcare Reality Check explains why it's thumbs down on the Atkins Diet.

www.mayo.edu/about.mayo_diet.html

"Ask the Mayo Dietician" contains an answer to the false "Mayo Diet" claims, plus lots of good advice on healthy eating and weight loss.

www.mayohealth.org/mayo

The Mayo Clinic Health Oasis offers a wealth of valuable health information. Click on "Nutrition" for articles, Q&As, self-assessment tools, tips, and solid facts about eating and weight loss.

www.nhlbisupport.com/cgi-bin/chd1/diet1.cgi

"Create-a-Diet Activity" will walk you through the process step by step.

www.phys.com

Click on "Nutrition," then go to "Diet Right" for reviews of diet books that are worth your time and money. Click on "Weight-loss" and then "The Diet Debunker" for a consumer's guide to the latest fad diets.

www.phys.com/self/eat

"Eat for Your Life" details healthy eating strategies for your 20s, 30s, and 40s.

www.thriveonline.com/eats/vitamins

This "Vitamin and Mineral Guide" will tell you what various micronutrients do, how much you need daily, where to get them in the food you eat, and what goes wrong if you have too little (or too much).

www.wellweb.com/nutri/fdaart.htm

The "FDA Guide to Dieting" is a no-nonsense article containing the facts on set point and a lot more about the science of weight loss and gain.

Exercise and fitness

www.acefitness.org

The American Council on Fitness web site is full of information on fitness. You can also find the name and contact information for ACE-certified personal trainers by city or zip code.

www.achillestrackclub.org

Achilles Track Club, a nonprofit organization that encourages people with disabilities to enjoy the benefits of running and walking, provides information about short- and long-distance recreational and competitive running and the locations of local chapters.

www.aerobics.com

"Exercise Gets Personal" is a customized program based on your answers to questions about your current fitness, lifestyle, and exercise preferences.

www.aoa.dhhs.gov/aoa/pages/agepages/exercise.html

"Feeling Fit for Life" offers fitness and exercise advice for seniors from the Administration on Aging.

www.drkoop.com/wellness/fitness

The "Fitness Center" area of this web site offers information, inspiration, facts, and ideas to help you get started.

www.drkoop.com/wellness/fitness/facts

"Exercise with Care" is a special section on exercise for people with disabilities and chronic illnesses.

www.learn2.com

Select the "Health and Fitness Channel" and type in "Stretch before exercising." You'll find an animated series of stretches that shows you exactly how to do it.

www.niddk.nih.gov/health/nutrit/pubs/walking.htm

"Walking … A Step in the Right Direction" is downloadable from the National Institute of Diabetes and Digestive and Kidney Diseases web site.

onhealth.com/fitness/in-depth/item/item,26183_1_.asp

Learn how to "Stretch Yourself at Work." The text will tell you why; the animations will show you how.

onhealth.com/fitness/in-depth/item/item,35662_1_1.asp

You'll find an excellent fitness assessment test at this site.

www.phys.com

"Burn more calories" asks a few easy questions and gives you a personalized analysis, complete with suggestions for what you can do to be more active.

www.phys.com/fitness/activities

"Sports & Activities" offers details on more than two dozen popular choices.

www.phys.com/fitness/analysis

Here's a fitness test you can perform at home.

www.phys.com/fitness/stretches

The "Stretching Guide" will show and tell you all you need to know to keep you supple for life.

www.phys.com/wsf/exdiet/plan.html

What's the Exercise Diet? All you want to eat in exchange for 60 minutes of varied activity 7 days a week. You'll find all the details here.

www.prevention.com/weight/buzz/980722.buzz.html

Find out "How to make exercise feel easier."

www.prevention.com/weight/buzz/more/html

"Body Buzz" is full of good ideas for overcoming exercise roadblocks.

www.prevention.com/weight/planner

Here's an extensive menu of workouts to mix and match.

www.prevention.com/weight/quiz

Take the "What's Your Workout Personality" quiz for an exercise routine that suits your personal style.

www.shapeup.org/fitness

Fill out the "Physical Activity Readiness Questionnaire" (PAR-Q) to find out if it's safe for you to begin to be more active. Then take a fitness test and read suggestions for appropriate activities for each level of fitness.

www.teleport.com/~walking/hiking.html

The "Walking & Hiking Homepage" is a treasure trove of information and links to treks, tours, clubs, and places to travel on foot in the United States and throughout the world.

www.thriveonline.com/shape/seniors/fit1.html

More ideas on fitness over 50.

Calculators and calorie counters

www.cyberdiet.com

A huge and comprehensive calorie counter can be found at this web site. The "Database of Foods" contains full nutritional info – including calories and grams of fat – on any quantity of anything you've ever dreamed of eating.

www.dawp.anet.com

The "Diet Analysis Web Page" will keep track of your daily intake and print out a chart or graph including calories, protein, and various vitamins and minerals. Includes lots of fast foods by brand.

www.4weightloss.com

"Keeping Track" will link you to several calorie counters and activity calculators. Two particularly useful calorie guides – "The Kitchen Counter" and "Fast Food Calculator" – can be found on this web site.

www.homearts.com:80/helpers/calculators/burnf1.htm

The "Burn Barometer" lists dozens of activities and the number of calories they burn.

www.ivillage.com/food/tools

The "Health Calculator" will ask a few personal questions and then figure out your carbohydrate, fat, and protein RDA and total daily calorie needs.

www.ivillage.com/tools/healthcalc

Here's a simple way to find out if you are within the normal range for your height, gender, and frame size.

www.phys.com

Click on "Calculators," then look under "Crunch Your Numbers" for "Health Risk." Punch in your numbers and it will figure out your waist-to-hip ratio (WHR). Look for "Phys Favorites" on the left side of the page and select "Snack-o-Matic." Make a selection from categories ranging from "sweet" or "salty" to "smooth" or "chunky," and find out the calorie and fat content of dozens of snacks. This cool tool will help you snack wisely.

www.phys.com/self/home.html

Choose an activity and enter the number of minutes you plan to do it, then click the calculator to find out how many calories you'll burn.

www.phys.com/weightloss

Play "The Snack Bandit" ("Tools & Quizzes") to find out how much activity a given food is worth. Then you decide if it's worth the trade.

www.primusweb.com/fitnesspartner

The "Fitness Partner Connection" lists dozens of activities ranging from gym and sports to daily life and occupational activities, along with the calorie burn you'll get according to your weight and the amount of time you do them.

www.shapeup.org

The "Cyberkitchen" will tell you how many calories you need each day.

www.thedietchannel.com

Click on "The Best Diet Analysis Tools on the Web" to find calorie needs calculators and much more.

www.thriveonline.com/cgibin/bmi.cgi

The calculator will not only figure out your BMI for you, but will also give you recommendations on what to do about the result.

Diaries

www.nhlbi.nih.gov/healh/public/heart

Here's a printable food and activity diary blank from the National Heart, Lung, and Blood Institute.

www.onhealth.com

Membership in this health "club" is free, and it includes an interactive "Diet and Fitness Journal."

www.thriveonline.com/weight/habits/week2.html

You'll find a printable food diary at this site.

Medical information

www.americanheart.org

The American Heart Association web site offers tips for heart-safe exercising for all ages and an interactive risk assessment of your personal heart health.

www.diabetes.org

The American Diabetes Association offers general information, a test to determine your own risk for developing this disease, and tips and information on exercise, nutrition, and other ways to prevent, treat, and live with diabetes.

jama.ama-assn.org/issues/v282n16

Find the special issue of the *Journal of the American Medical Association* devoted to weight and weight loss at this site.

www.niddk.nih.gov/health/pubs/gastsurg.htm

You'll find an online pamphlet about stomach surgery from the National Institute of Diabetes and Digestive and Kidney Diseases at this site.

Government sites

odphp.osophs.dhhs.gov/pubs/hp2000/

The Healthy People 2000 web site features information about national fitness goals, including the year 2010 targets.

vm.cfsan.fda.gov/~DMS/aems.html

The FDA's Center for Food Safety and Applied Nutrition, Office of Special Nutritionals, web site will tell you everything you want to know about potentially unpleasant or dangerous side effects of over-the-counter weight-loss and other diet supplements. Searchable by ingredient or product name.

warp.nal.usda.gov:80/fnic/dga

The U.S. Department of Agriculture's Food and Nutrition Information Center web site features the latest "Dietary Guidelines for Americans," lots of solid information about nutrition, and useful links to other sites.

www.usda.gov/cnpp
www.niddk.nih.gov
www.nhlbi.nih.gov/health/pubs

The Center for Nutrition Policy and Promotion, the National Institute of Diabetes and Digestive and Kidney Diseases, and the National Heart, Lung, and Blood Institute are three federal agencies that offer solid information on diet and exercise and useful links.

Support and advice

www.aabainc.org

The American Anorexia Bulimia Association web site offers information, support, and referral networks for people suffering from eating disorders.

boards.excite.com

One of many web portals hosting online message boards. Click on "Health" and then "Diet and Nutrition" or "Exercise and Fitness" when you need support.

www.eatright.org

The American Dietetic Association web site will tell you what dieticians do and help you find a registered dietician in your area.

www.magazine-rack.com

This web site contains a large selection of online magazines organized by subject.

www.overeatersanonymous.org

Find out about Overeaters Anonymous and take a quiz to help you determine if you are an overeater.

www.thriveonline.com

Click on "Weight Management," then "Programs & Products" for information on commercial weight-loss programs. There's also a message board with discussions about various diet plans, programs, and products.

www.tops.org

Find out about Take Off Pounds Sensibly (TOPS), information about its philosophy and approach to weight loss, and how to sign up.

A simple glossary

Aerobic In the presence of oxygen; used to describe any exercise or sustained physical activity that increases supply of oxygen to muscles and improves cardiovascular fitness. *Compare to* Anaerobic.

Amino acid One of 80 organic compounds that form proteins in humans and other living things; 20 are necessary for human growth and development; the body makes some (called nonessential amino acids), but others must be supplied by food (called essential amino acids).

Anaerobic Without oxygen; used to describe activity that does not increase supply of oxygen to muscles or improve cardiovascular fitness; short bursts of effort are fueled by stored energy. *Compare to* Aerobic.

Anemia Deficiency or defect in oxygen-carrying red blood cells as a result of one of many factors; symptoms include fatigue and weakness.

Angina Chest pain, especially during exercise or exertion, resulting from insufficient blood and oxygen supply to the heart; often a symptom of coronary artery disease.

Anorexia nervosa Potentially life-threatening eating disorder, most common in teenage girls, characterized by extreme food avoidance and dangerously subnormal weight.

Antioxidant Any substance that inhibits or prevents oxidation, a process of decay that includes rusting (in metals) and spoilage (in some foods), and is believed to be involved in some disease processes.

Artery Type of blood vessel that carries oxygen-rich blood from the lungs to the entire body.

Atherosclerosis Narrowing of arteries as a result of cholesterol deposits on their inner walls; consequences include angina, coronary artery disease, heart attack, and stroke.

Basal metabolism Amount of energy used for basic body processes, excluding voluntary physical activity.

Beta carotene Yellow to red pigment found in many foods and converted to vitamin A by the liver; valued for its antioxidant properties.

Binge eating Episodes of uncontrolled eating, usually of large quantities; sign of an eating disorder.

BMR Basal (or basic) metabolic rate; rate at which the body performs basal metabolism.

Body dysphoria Psychological condition in which a person has a false sense of his or her own body, often feeling fat when the opposite is true; a common feature of anorexia nervosa.

Body mass index (BMI) Formula used to estimate proportion of the body that consists of fat: weight (kg) ÷ height^2 (m).

Bulimia An eating disorder in which episodes of binge eating are followed by purging, through vomiting and abuse of laxatives and enemas.

Calorie Unit of heat measurement; amount of energy needed to raise temperature of 1 gram of water 1 degree Celsius; used to measure amount of energy available in food and used by activity.

Calorie density Ratio between a given food's weight and its calorie content.

Carbohydrate One of the three basic nutrient types; complex carbohydrates are starches, simple carbohydrates are sugars; body's main source of energy.

Cardiorespiratory Combined function of heart and lungs working together to pump oxygenated blood.

Cardiovascular An umbrella word referring to the heart and blood vessels.

Cellulite Layperson's term for puckery fat visible beneath skin; contrary to popular myth, it is no different from any other stored fat in the body.

Cellulose Also called fiber; highly complex carbohydrate indigestible by humans; can be soluble or insoluble in water.

Cholesterol Fatty substance produced by the liver (endogenous) and present in some foods (exogenous). In normal amounts, essential for many body processes, including producing hormones.

In excess, can cause atherosclerosis. *See also* HDL, LDL, Triglyceride.

Chromium picolinate   Synthetic form of chromium, an essential trace mineral abundantly available in food; sold in health food stores as a cholesterol-lowering and metabolism-boosting agent; excess amounts cause flushing, nervousness, and palpitations, and iron deficiency.

Clinical nutritionist   Professional trained in nutrition science with doctoral-level training (MD or PhD).

Coronary arteries   Arteries located on the outside wall of the heart that supply blood to the heart muscle itself.

Coronary artery disease (CAD)   Narrowing of the arteries that supply blood to the heart muscles; a major cause of heart attacks.

Diabetes   Metabolic disorder in which the body does not make enough insulin or cannot use it effectively. Type 1 diabetes is a relatively rare autoimmune disease. Type 2 diabetes is a very common disease; risk factors include overweight, high cholesterol, and lack of exercise; complications include blindness, loss of limbs, kidney failure, and cardiovascular disease.

Diastolic   Blood pressure when heart muscle relaxes; diastolic pressure is the second, lower, number in any blood pressure reading, e.g., 120/80. *Compare to* Systolic.

Dietitian   Licensed professional with college- or graduate-level education in nutrition science. An American Dietetic Association (ADA) registered dietitian (RD) license requires a bachelor's degree; a dietetic technician, registered (DTR) license requires a two-year associate's degree.

Diverticulitis   Painful condition resulting when small pouches (diverticula) that form in colon wall are clogged with feces and become inflamed.

Eating disorder   Psychological illness in which food is abused, through excessive eating (compulsive eating), bingeing and purging (bulimia), or extreme food denial (anorexia nervosa).

Emetic   Vomit inducer.

Endogenous   Literally "coming from within." Refers to a substance the body makes rather than taking it in from an outside source. *Compare to* Exogenous.

Endurance   Ability to sustain physical activity; also called cardiovascular, cardiorespiratory, or aerobic fitness.

Ephedra   An herbal extract; also called Ma huang; sold in health food stores as a weight-loss supplement; suppresses appetite by stimulating the nervous system and thyroid gland; side effects include numbness in hands and feet, blood pressure elevation, nervousness, and palpitations.

Exogenous   Literally "coming from outside." Refers to a substance taken into the body from an outside source. *Compare to* Endogenous.

Fat   Also called lipid; non-water-soluble substance used by body for energy, vitamin transport, normal growth and development, and to build and maintain many body systems. *See also* Saturated fat, Unsaturated fat.

Fatty acid   A molecular component of fat; main product of fat metabolism; not soluble in water.

FDA   US Food and Drug Administration, federal agency in charge of regulating safety and effectiveness of prescription drugs.

Fitness   Ability of body to do work required of it; main components are endurance, flexibility, and strength.

Flexibility   Also referred to as range of motion; ability to bend and stretch easily; measure of fitness of muscles, joints, and connective tissue.

Food pyramid   Graphic guide to the currently recommended balanced diet.

Functional food   An edible product found in the grocery store that has medicinal properties, such as the ability to lower cholesterol.

Gastric bypass   Surgical procedure sometimes used in morbidly obese patients in which food is routed past all or a portion of the stomach in an effort to limit caloric intake.

Gastric restriction   Surgical procedure sometimes used in morbidly obese patients in which a portion of the stomach is closed off in an effort to limit caloric intake.

Glucomannan   Indigestible bulking agent marketed as a diet aid; can cause dangerous bowel obstruction.

Glucose   A simple sugar; main breakdown product of carbohydrate metabolism.

Glycogen   Form in which glucose is stored by body.

HDL   High-density lipoprotein; a type of cholesterol that protects against development of atherosclerosis; the "good" cholesterol.

High blood pressure   *see* Hypertension.

Hypertension   Also called high blood pressure; condition in which pressure of blood pumped through arteries is consistently higher than normal; pressure in excess of 140/90.

Hyperthyroidism   Overactivity of the thyroid gland; symptoms include weight loss, appetite increase, nervousness and tremor, insomnia, diarrhea, bulging eyes, racing heartbeat, excessive sweating, and heat intolerance, due to increased metabolic rate.

Hypothalamus   Area of brain thought to control appetite.

Hypothyroidism   Underactivity of the thyroid gland; symptoms include weight gain, sluggishness, fatigue.

Insulin   Hormone that converts sugar, starches, and other foods to energy; in diabetes, the body does not make enough insulin or cannot use it effectively.

Intensity   Relative term indicating how hard the heart works during any activity; minimal intensity is at lower end of the target heart rate zone, maximal intensity at upper end of the zone.

Interval training   Method of intensifying an aerobic workout by increasing speed to increase heart rate in measured bursts; typically, a one-minute push every three to five minutes.

Ketogenic   Anything that causes ketosis; high-protein diets are ketogenic.

Ketone   A chemical byproduct of incomplete fat metabolism.

Ketosis   Accumulation of ketones as a consequence of incomplete metabolism of fatty acids; occurs when carbohydrates are deficient or cannot be used because of a metabolic disorder.

LDL   Low-density lipoprotein; a type of cholesterol that leaves deposits on artery walls, leading to atherosclerosis; the "bad" cholesterol.

Liposuction   Cosmetic surgical procedure in which fat deposits under the skin are liquefied and suctioned out through a narrow tube.

Low-impact aerobics   A type of exercise performed with one foot always in contact with the floor as a means of reducing shock to the joints that may occur with jumping jacks and other "high-impact" movements. Like any aerobic exercise, it aims to raise the heart rate into the target zone to improve cardiovascular fitness.

Maximum heart rate (MHR)   Theoretical upper limit of number of times per minute the human heart can beat; in general, MHR decreases with age.

Metabolism   All of the chemical and physical processes by which the body breaks down, converts, and uses food, gases, and other substances.

Night eating syndrome (NES)   Type of eating disorder, possibly due to a defect in brain chemistry, in which a person eats a lot at bedtime and even awakens at night to eat; obesity and insomnia are symptoms.

Nutritionist   Advisor on food and nutrition; does not require or imply specialized education or licensing. *Compare to* Dietician, Clinical nutritionist.

Obesity   Weight in excess of 20 percent of standard for height, age, and gender; body mass index (BMI) of 30 or greater.

Olestra   A synthetic fat that cannot be absorbed by the body and thus provides no calories.

Orlistat   A prescription fat-blocker marketed under the name Xenical.

Physiological   Related to body functions.

Placebo   Dummy pill, usually made of sugar, that is used in research trials to test the effectiveness of a medication; placebo is used as the "control" part of an experiment.

Proteins Complex molecular compounds found in plant and animal foods; essential for building and maintaining muscles and other tissues; supply heat and energy.

Rep Repetition; number of times an action, such as lifting a weight, is repeated.

Resting heart rate (RHR) Number of times per minute an individual's heart beats while inactive.

Saturated fat Found in animal products, including meat and dairy, coconut and palm oils; solid at room temperature due to extra hydrogen atoms; raises levels of LDL cholesterol in the blood.

Set A group of reps, or repetitions; 8 to 12 reps are usually considered a set; used for counting during exercise.

Set point Theoretical personal "ideal" weight predetermined by the hypothalamus. Scientists do not yet fully understand the exact details of this mechanism.

Sprain Injury to one of the ligaments that connect bone to bone; symptoms include sharp pain, usually followed by stiffness, tenderness, and swelling.

Stamina Vigor, endurance; capacity to withstand fatigue or disease.

Strain Also called "pulled muscle," or "charley horse." Overstretched or torn muscle fiber due to sudden movement; symptoms include pain, stiffness, and swelling.

Strength Ability of muscles to exert force to push, pull, or lift; measure of muscular fitness.

Stroke Damage to the brain due to interruption in blood supply; ischemic stroke occurs when the flow of blood to the brain is blocked; hemorrhagic stroke occurs when there is bleeding in the brain.

Systolic Blood pressure when the heart muscle contracts; systolic pressure is the first, higher, number in any blood pressure reading, e.g., 120/80. *Compare to* Diastolic.

Target heart rate (THR) Percentage of an individual's maximum heart rate (MHR) designated as a measure of exercise intensity.

Thyroid Butterfly-shaped gland that wraps around the windpipe; secretes hormones that regulate metabolism. *See also* Hyperthyroidism, Hypothyroidism.

Trans fat Unsaturated fat that has been hydrogenated, a process by which hydrogen atoms are added to retard spoilage and make the fat solidify at room temperature; trans fats raise LDL and lower HDL levels, increasing risk of heart disease.

Triglyceride A lipid, or fatty substance, found in blood; high levels contribute to atherosclerosis and coronary artery disease.

Unsaturated fat Found in vegetables, seeds, and fish; liquid at room temperature. Can be monounsaturated or polyunsaturated; thought to lower LDL cholesterol levels.

USDA U.S. Department of Agriculture; federal agency that issues dietary guidelines, including the food pyramid, and maintains a database of the nutritional content of foods, including calorie counts.

Vein Type of blood vessel that carries oxygen-depleted blood back to the lungs.

Waist-to-hip ratio (WHR) Waist measurement divided by hip measurement; WHR for women should be .8 or less, for men .95 or less.

Weight cycling Also called yo-yo dieting; repeated loss and gain of weight through successive, but not successful, dieting.

Index

Acknowledgments

Cooling Brown would like to thank Alison Bolus and Janet Swarbrick for their editorial assistance, and Barry Robson for illustrating the dogs, and bringing them so vividly to life.

Index
Hilary Bird.

Picture credits
Photodisc: 16–17, 18–19, 21, 22, 35, 42, 53, 54, 56, 61tl, 68, 69, 70, 94, 105, 110, 125, 126, 128, 129, 130, 136, 138, 145, 150br, 152, 155tl, 157br, 159, 166, 171, 172, 182, 183tr, 186, 188, 190, 195, 196, 200, 201, 203, 206, 207, 208, 212, 216, 217, 218, 224, 237, 239, 249, 252, 253, 254, 257, 258, 260, 266, 269tr, 274, 275, 277br, 278, 284, 285, 287, 288, 289, 291, 292, 293, 297, 300, 301, 303, 308, 312, 314, 317, 318, 319, 320tr, 322br, 323, 324, 325, 326, 333, 334, 336, 340, 341.
The Stock Market Photo Agency Inc: 232 Jon Feingersh, 88 and 264 Michael Keller, 220 and 282 Rob Lewine, 250 Jose L. Pelaez Inc., 118 and 205 Steve Prezant, 100 Ariel Skelley, 38, 298 and 328 unidentified, 2 David Woods.

Additional photography
Andy Crawford, Philip Dowell, Steve Gorton, Paul Harris, Dave King, Ian O'Leary, Kevin Mallett, Ranald Mckechnie, Tracy Morgan, David Murray, Stephen Oliver, Roger Phillips, Susanna Price, Tim Ridley, Kim Sayer, Jules Selmes, Jane Stockman, Clive Streeter, Colin Walton, Matthew Ward, Andrew Whittuck, Philip Wilkins.